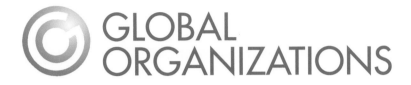

GLOBAL ORGANIZATIONS

The World Health Organization

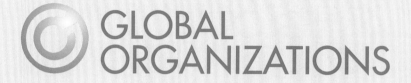

GLOBAL ORGANIZATIONS

The African Union

The Arab League

The Association of Southeast Asian Nations

The Caribbean Community

The European Union

The International Atomic Energy Agency

The Organization of American States

The Organization of the Petroleum
Exporting Countries

The United Nations

The United Nations Children's Fund

The World Bank and
the International Monetary Fund

The World Health Organization

The World Trade Organization

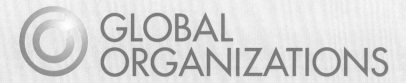

GLOBAL
ORGANIZATIONS

The World Health Organization

G. S. Prentzas

Series Editor
Peggy Kahn
University of Michigan–Flint

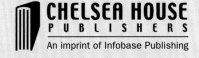

CHELSEA HOUSE
PUBLISHERS
An imprint of Infobase Publishing

The World Health Organization

Copyright © 2009 by Infobase Publishing

All rights reserved. No part of this book may be reproduced or utilized in any form or by any means, electronic or mechanical, including photocopying, recording, or by any information storage or retrieval systems, without permission in writing from the publisher. For information contact:

Chelsea House
An imprint of Infobase Publishing
132 West 31st Street
New York NY 10001

Library of Congress Cataloging-in-Publication Data
Prentzas, G. S.
The World Health Organization / G.S. Prentzas.
      p. cm. — (Global organizations)
Includes bibliographical references and index.
ISBN 978-0-7910-9839-4 (hardcover)
1. World Health Organization. I. Title. II. Series.

RA8.P74 2009
362.1—dc22   2009000321

Chelsea House books are available at special discounts when purchased in bulk quantities for businesses, associations, institutions, or sales promotions. Please call our Special Sales Department in New York at (212) 967-8800 or (800) 322-8755.

You can find Chelsea House on the World Wide Web at http://www.chelseahouse.com

Series design by Erik Lindstrom
Cover design by Ben Peterson

Printed in the United States of America

Bang KT 10 9 8 7 6 5 4 3 2 1

This book is printed on acid-free paper.

All links and Web addresses were checked and verified to be correct at the time of publication. Because of the dynamic nature of the Web, some addresses and links may have changed since publication and may no longer be valid.

CONTENTS

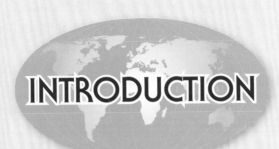

INTRODUCTION

Outbreak!

IN FEBRUARY 2003, A HOSPITAL IN HANOI, VIETNAM, TRANS-ferred a patient to a hospital in Hong Kong, China. The symptoms of the patient, Johnny Chen, included fever, weakness, a dry cough, and respiratory problems. The 46-year-old American businessman's condition quickly worsened. Within a few days, health-care workers at the Hong Kong hospital began to get sick. They had the same symptoms as Chen. The Hanoi hospital where Chen first sought care reported that a similar outbreak was racing through its facility. On March 13, Chen died of an unknown type of pneumonia.

Medical experts first believed that the disease that killed Chen was a type of bird flu. A month earlier, two people in Hong Kong had been diagnosed with a rare form of influenza found in birds. One had died. Scientists had already discovered that humans could sometimes contract flu viruses that afflict birds. In 1997, a deadly strain of flu that had jumped from birds to humans infected 18 people in Hong Kong, killing 6.

Medical tests on the patients in the Hong Kong and Hanoi hospitals showed that the new deadly disease was not caused by a virus or bacteria associated with bird flu or any other known type of influenza. Researchers realized that this was a new type of respiratory disease. They gave it a name: severe acute respiratory syndrome (SARS).

To help doctors diagnose the disease, health officials quickly identified and distributed a list of the symptoms of SARS. The disease begins with a high fever (temperature exceeding 100.4° F [38.0° C]). Other symptoms then occur, including headache, body aches, and an overall feeling of discomfort. Some patients also have mild respiratory symptoms. Two to seven days later, many SARS patients develop a dry cough. Most patients eventually develop pneumonia, the disease that killed Chen, the first known victim.

Because SARS appeared to spread so quickly and easily, researchers originally thought that it was passed from person to person by close contact. They would later agree that an infected person could transmit SARS through coughing or sneezing. When a person with SARS coughs or sneezes, she or he sends thousands of droplets into the air. These droplets can travel up to 3 feet (0.9 meters). People nearby can be infected if the droplets land on the mucous membranes of their mouth, nose, or eyes. People can also become infected with SARS by touching the droplets and then touching their mouth, nose, or eyes. Researchers believe that SARS can spread through the air in other ways yet undiscovered.

With the identification of SARS, the twenty-first century's first severe infectious disease had arrived. (An infectious disease is spread, often person to person, by germs entering the body.) New SARS cases began to multiply. The disease spread to at least 15 countries, including Canada, Germany, Singapore, and the United States. In Canada, two Toronto hospitals had to turn away new patients to help prevent the disease from spreading further. Health officials in Hong Kong placed an entire apartment building under a quarantine, or medical isolation.

Researchers tried to trace the disease back to its origins. They determined that a 72-year-old man from Beijing, China, was one of the first people to contract SARS. He took at least one plane trip before he began to experience any symptoms. During that trip, he probably infected as many as 22 passengers. Many of these people took planes to other countries, spreading the disease. The movement of these passengers made it very difficult for health officials to track down the virus and quarantine those who might pass it on. They discovered that one passenger had taken seven international flights before SARS symptoms appeared. He had traveled throughout Europe and Asia before seeking medical care.

On April 16, 2003, the World Health Organization (WHO) announced that several laboratories had discovered and confirmed the cause of SARS. The respiratory disease is caused by a coronavirus now known as SARS-associated coronavirus (SARS-CoV). (The name *coronavirus* comes from the spikes that stick out of the virus's surface; *corona* is the Latin word for "crown.") The virus damages alveoli, the tiny air-filled sacs in the lungs where oxygen and carbon dioxide are exchanged between the lungs and the bloodstream. SARS can lead to death as a result of progressive respiratory failure.

Over the next few months, SARS spread to 30 countries in Asia, Europe, North America, and South America. In May 2003, more than 180 new infections were being reported daily. Health officials around the world scrambled to contain the outbreak. Luckily, SARS proved to be less infectious than officials first believed. From 2003 to 2005, about 8,500 people worldwide became sick with SARS. Of these, 812 died. About 20 percent of those infected were health-care workers exposed to patients with SARS. Among the early victims was Dr. Carlo

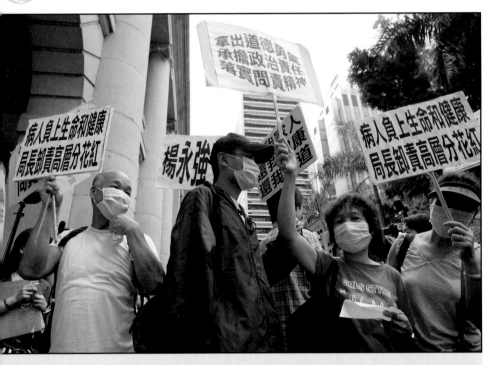

Between November 2002 and July 2003, SARS spread from Guangdong province in China to some 37 countries around the world, causing worldwide panic. WHO estimates that SARS caused more than 8,000 infected cases and more than 700 deaths. In June 2004, recovered SARS patients and family members (shown above) protested the handling of the outbreak by the Chinese government, which eventually admitted to underreporting the number of SARS cases.

Urbani, a WHO doctor in Vietnam. He had examined Johnny Chen at the hospital in Hanoi and concluded that he was suffering from some unknown disease. Urbani had been the person who first brought SARS to the attention of the world's health community.

By 2005, WHO reported that SARS had been stamped out, at least for the time being. Although this century's first new infectious disease did not result in a devastating outbreak, it did point out that new microbial threats to human health can seemingly arise out of nowhere. In the past 25 years, medical researchers have identified more than 30 new diseases. The SARS outbreak underscored the growing importance in an increasingly globalized world of improving international public health cooperation to prevent the spread of infectious diseases.

In July 2003, Dr. Gro Harlem Brundtland, then the director-general of WHO, noted:

> SARS is a warning. SARS pushed even the most advanced public-health systems to the breaking point. Those protections held, but just barely. Next time, we may not be so lucky. We have an opportunity now, and we see the need clearly, to rebuild our public-health protections. They will be needed for the next global outbreak, if it is SARS or another new infection.[1]

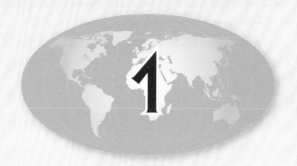

Introduction to the World Health Organization

WHEN WORLD WAR II ENDED IN 1945, MANY CITIES IN EUROPE and Japan lay in ruins. Battles had been fought in Europe, Africa, and Asia and at sea. During the six-year global conflict, warfare had killed more than 50 million soldiers and civilians. Countless farms, factories, and businesses had been destroyed. Uncontrolled infectious diseases—such as smallpox, measles, and tuberculosis—swept through many parts of the world. Millions of people—many of them now without homes—desperately needed health care to heal their wounds or to treat illnesses brought on by years of poverty, hunger, and medical neglect.

This was the state of the world in 1946 when the United Nations (UN) invited public health experts from around the world to a conference in New York City. (One year earlier, the nations of the world had joined together to create the UN, an

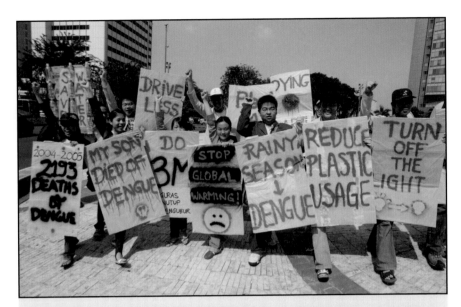

Since 1950, April 7 has been celebrated annually as World Health Day, marking the founding day of WHO. Every year World Health Day is used as an opportunity to highlight a priority area of concern to global health. In 2008, the theme was "protecting health from climate change," which focused on helping the global community to be better prepared to cope with climate-related health challenges worldwide.

international organization devoted to providing peace and security for all countries.) At the conference, the delegates worked to establish a global health organization known as the World Health Organization (WHO).

In drafting a constitution to provide the structure and basic principles of the new organization, the public-health experts agreed on a bold goal for WHO. Article I of the constitution proclaimed that the organization's mission would be "the attainment by all peoples of the highest possible level of health." The constitution defined *health* as "not merely the absence of disease or infirmity" but "a state of complete physical, mental, and social well-being."[2] This groundbreaking goal grew out of two fundamental ideas: that every nation has a duty to protect the health of its citizens and that nations can work together to prevent the spread of dangerous diseases. WHO's constitution came into force on April 7, 1948. The seventh day of April is now celebrated as World Health Day.

ERADICATING SMALLPOX: A WHO SUCCESS STORY

One of the World Health Organization's proudest achievements has been the eradication of smallpox. So far, it is the only major infectious disease ever to have been stamped out.

Smallpox is a deadly and highly contagious disease caused by a virus. There are two main types of smallpox. *Variola major* is the far more serious form. It killed one-third to one-half of all those who were infected. *Variola minor* is the much less deadly type, killing less than 2 percent of people who contracted it. Smallpox left its mark on survivors. More than two-thirds suffered from permanent, deep-pitted scars, known as pockmarks, on the face and other parts of the body. Smallpox also caused blindness in many cases.

The smallpox virus spread easily from one person to another through face-to-face transmission. When sufferers coughed, they released huge amounts of virus particles into the air. Clothing and bedding infected with the virus could also spread smallpox. There is no effective medical treatment.

Beginning as early as 10,000 B.C., smallpox epidemics swept across continents. The disease killed millions and affected the course of human history. Epidemics left countries unable to defend themselves against their enemies and killed powerful world leaders. Egyptian pharaoh Ramses V, Incan emperor Huayna Capac, King Louis XV of France, and other leaders died from smallpox. U.S. presidents George Washington and Abraham Lincoln and Soviet premier Joseph Stalin all survived the disease.

Today, WHO has 193 member countries. Its membership includes every nation in the UN except Liechtenstein, plus two small, non-UN nations (Niue and the Cook Islands). WHO is a specialized agency of the United Nations. It governs itself, but the UN's Economic and Social Council oversees its activi-

In 1798, British doctor Edward Jenner discovered that injecting patients with a small amount of the cowpox virus created a natural immunity to smallpox. Cowpox is in the same virus family as smallpox, but it is rarely dangerous. Despite the development of Jenner's vaccine, hundreds of thousands of people continued to die from smallpox. Most lived in poor countries or remote areas of wealthier countries. In the early 1950s—a century and a half after the smallpox vaccination became available—an estimated 50 million cases of smallpox still occurred worldwide each year. As methodical smallpox vaccination programs spread, however, cases plunged to about 10 million a year by the mid-1960s. Smallpox remained dangerous. It killed about 25 percent of its victims and scarred or blinded most survivors.

WHO began to coordinate a global smallpox vaccination program in 1967. The program successfully provided vaccinations for at-risk populations around the world. The last known natural case of smallpox occurred in the African country of Somalia in 1977. Since then, the only known smallpox cases were caused by a 1978 accident in an English medical laboratory. One of the two lab workers infected in that incident died. On May 8, 1980, during its annual World Health Assembly, WHO declared that smallpox had been eradicated.

In the event of a future outbreak, small stockpiles of smallpox vaccine are held in high-security labs in Russia and the United States.

ties. Although the people who wrote WHO's constitution could not have foreseen many of the twenty-first century's health challenges, they created an organization that remains critically important to the health and welfare of humankind.

Advances in medical science in the twentieth century produced vaccines and treatments for a wide range of diseases. Recent research involving human stem cells and new discoveries in molecular biology, including DNA cloning and the Human Genome Project, offer hope that more diseases can be controlled or eliminated. Many important victories in the ongoing struggle against disease have been won. WHO has spearheaded efforts resulting in the eradication, or elimination, of smallpox. Polio and Guinea worm disease have almost been eradicated. Polio is a disease that can cause paralysis by attacking the spinal cord. Guinea worm disease, which is found mostly in Africa, is caused by microscopic worm larvae that enter the human body when a person drinks contaminated water. (Once inside the body, the threadlike parasite can grow up to 3 feet [0.9 meters] in length!).

Measles, known for its distinctive red skin rash, may be the next highly contagious disease to be eradicated. In 1980, measles killed more than 5 million children. From 2000 to 2006, WHO supported a project that vaccinated an estimated 478 million children in 46 high-risk countries. In 2006, an estimated 242,000 people of all ages died from measles, a two-thirds drop from 2000. In Africa, measles cases and deaths plunged 91 percent over those seven years.

Despite these successes, however, WHO's goal of advancing good health care worldwide remains a daunting one. More than half of the world's population lives in developing countries. (Developing countries are also known as less-developed, or low-income, countries.) More than 100 of the world's 195 countries are considered to be developing countries. In these nations, insufficient nutrition, unsafe drinking water, and poor sanitation combine to create high rates of disease and death. Worldwide, more than 2.5 billion people live on less than $2 a day. Few poor people can afford health care. Many live far from health-care services.

Children in many poor families suffer from malnutrition, which stunts their physical development, impairs their ability to learn, and weakens their immune systems. (The immune system is the body's defense system that protects against viruses, bacteria, and other invaders.) Each year, nearly 10 million children in developing countries die before they reach their fifth birthday. Acquired immune deficiency syndrome (AIDS), malaria, respiratory infections, and intestinal diseases remain major killers of children and adults in the developing world.

More than 6 billion people now live on Earth. By 2100, the population may reach 10 billion. Research has shown that as places become more heavily populated, deadly diseases like cholera and tuberculosis spread more quickly and easily. Citizens of all nations remain at risk of contracting long-established diseases and newer, even more dangerous diseases. Modern improvements in transportation and technology have increased the flow of information and people between countries. This trend, known as globalization, will continue to change the ways countries connect with one another. This increasing connectivity also allows diseases to spread around the world. Health has become a responsibility shared by all nations, rich and poor. It requires fair, universal access to essential health care and a united defense against highly contagious diseases that can threaten all nations.

WHO WORKS TO ENSURE GOOD HEALTH

As a specialized agency of the United Nations, WHO is an intergovernmental organization. Intergovernmental organizations are permanent international associations focused on specific global issues. Their memberships are made up of countries. More than 300 intergovernmental organizations operate in the world, including such notable groups as the UN, the European Union, and the World Trade Organization.

The World Health Assembly is WHO's decision-making body. Each May, delegations from all 193 member nations meet in Geneva, Switzerland. At this conference, delegates vote on many resolutions. These resolutions deal with such matters as establishing health programs, determining the organization's policies, or approving partnerships with other organizations. WHO's Executive Board writes the resolutions and presents them to the delegates. The Executive Board has 34 members, all of whom are experts in the public health field. Delegates at the World Health Assembly elect these board members, who serve three-year terms. Delegates also select WHO's director-general, who serves for five years. The director-general approves the budgets for WHO programs and also supervises the work of the organization's permanent staff. About 8,000 employees, health experts, and other staff members work at WHO headquarters in Geneva, in 6 regional offices, and in 147 countries.

WHO carries out its mission by providing leadership on a wide range of global health issues. It influences public health research worldwide, from the development of vaccines to the improvement of sanitation practices. The organization promotes cooperation between scientists and health researchers. Based on scientific evidence, it develops health-policy recommendations for nations to adopt. WHO monitors and assesses global health trends. It assists nations in addressing global health problems jointly and helps governments in developing countries improve their health services. WHO works with many partners, including other UN agencies (like UNICEF—the United Nations Children's Fund), nongovernmental organizations (like the Carter Center), and private corporations (like drug companies).

These partnerships help WHO achieve its goal of improving the well-being of people around the world. For example, WHO responded to a 2002 outbreak of a rare type of meningitis, a fatal disease of the thin covering of the brain or spinal cord, in the African country of Burkina Faso. WHO staff members worked closely with a large pharmaceutical company to develop a new vaccine. The vaccine was tested and approved in record time. WHO negotiated with the company to lower the

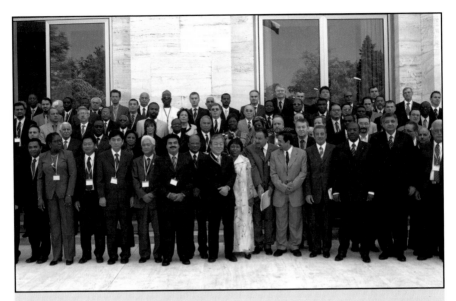

Members of the 57th World Health Assembly pose for a group photo during the annual meeting of the 193 member states in May 2004. The meeting focused on several health topics, including HIV/AIDS, reproductive health, road safety, dietary habits, and patterns of physical activity.

cost of the vaccine to less than a dollar per injection, a price that the government of Burkina Faso could afford.

The work did not end there. A more effective, low-cost meningitis vaccine was scheduled to be introduced in 2009. With support from WHO, the Meningitis Vaccine Project signed a deal with the Serum Institute of India to produce 25 million doses of vaccine for African countries over a period of 10 years. The new vaccine costs 40 cents. Kader Kondé, the vaccine project's representative working in WHO's office in Burkina Faso, noted, "The advantage of the new vaccine is that it is going to be affordable."[3]

In carrying out its mission, WHO's global health programs focus on several key areas:

- prevention of diseases through vaccines and immunization

- treatment of diseases
- health care for mothers and children in developing countries
- nutrition
- sanitation, including safe drinking water and proper disposal of human waste

WHO plays a major role in helping people in all countries live safer and healthier lives. It helps nations strengthen their health-care systems, which include national health ministries, hospitals, clinics, and other medical facilities. WHO also helps developing nations create programs to increase their national wealth and improve the well-being of their citizens. It advises wealthy, developed countries on the health threats to their citizens, such as chronic diseases. These diseases—like stroke, heart disease, cancer, obesity, diabetes, and asthma—are the leading killers of people in developed countries. WHO improves global health security through immunizations, treatment, and speedy responses to outbreaks of diseases. It publishes reliable public health information and research.

The importance of WHO's role is made clear by Winnie Mpanju, a doctor from Tanzania who works in WHO's headquarters:

Having worked with global and regional health organizations, national health systems, training institutions, health providers, and donors, I'm convinced that WHO's neutral and convening role is indispensable in addressing health priorities, especially among the poor and underprivileged. From our policy guidelines and standard setting to our work with other UN agencies and partners—all our work at HQ must add value in countries and benefit the people we serve. That is why we are here, plain and simple.[4]

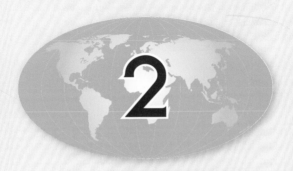

The Rise of International Public Health

THE ORIGINS OF THE WORLD HEALTH ORGANIZATION CAN BE traced back to international sanitary conferences that began in the eighteenth century and to international health organizations founded in the early twentieth century. International cooperation on health issues began about 700 years ago. In the fourteenth century, trade and commerce between countries and continents began to increase as people developed ways to build ships that could travel farther. The number of goods and people moving around the globe rose rapidly. Deadly diseases also began to spread more quickly worldwide.

Europeans made the first efforts at modern public health policy. Beginning in the fourteenth century, many European cities and countries passed laws to prevent the spread of disease. At that time, people did not know what caused diseases.

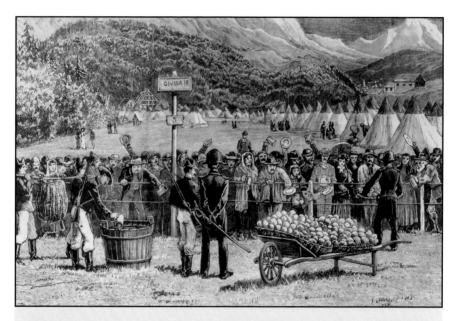

Although cholera is no longer considered a major global health threat, the disease still heavily affects less developed countries due to a lack of clean drinking water. Cholera, which spread by trade routes, has caused millions of deaths due to outbreaks in India, Russia, Western Europe, and North America since 1816. In this drawing, victims of the 1884 cholera epidemic are waiting to be fed by soldiers in a quarantine camp on the Franco-Italian border.

They observed that a disease would often spread from house to house and from village to village. People came to believe that if they touched a sick person—or even something that belonged to the person—they could catch the disease.

The government of Venice was the first to take action to stop the spread of disease. At the time, it was a powerful city-state. Located on the Adriatic Sea in what is now Italy, Venice had become a major shipping port on the trade routes between Europe and Asia and Africa. Each year, its harbor welcomed hundreds of ships from abroad. These ships brought trade goods and travelers, as well as diseases that had never been seen before in Europe. Because Europeans had not built up natural immunity to these diseases, outbreaks sometimes dispersed quickly.

To prevent diseases from these faraway lands from infecting its citizens, the government of Venice adopted a ground-breaking law. It required ships from abroad to anchor at an island outside of the city. The ship had to stay there for 40 days before it was allowed to proceed to Venice's docks to unload passengers and goods. Authorities in Venice believed that within 40 days a person infected with a contagious disease would either be cured or die. This 40-day period was known as a *quarantena*, from the Italian word *quaranta* ("40"). The law also required that cargo either be treated with smoke or be exposed to sunlight. The authorities believed that these methods made the cargo safe to unload.

Venice's practice of quarentena appeared to lessen disease among the city's population. Other countries began to isolate arriving ships. In the English language, the practice became known as a *quarantine*. Isolating ships from abroad for a set number of days, however, did not stop epidemics. Such diseases as bubonic plague and typhus still ravaged countries throughout the world. At the time, no one knew that a rat on a ship or lice hidden in a traveler's clothing might be carrying the microorganisms that cause these diseases. Having no better way to protect public health, governments continued to enforce quarantines until the nineteenth century.

INTERNATIONAL COOPERATION

During the early 1800s, the Industrial Revolution spread throughout Europe and the United States. The development of scientific knowledge, machinery, and larger businesses changed the economic, social, and political conditions of many countries. Goods that had been made in small workshops and homes for centuries by craftsmen began to be mass-produced in factories by workers. Cities grew rapidly as people moved from the countryside to find jobs in factories.

Trade and travel boomed as newfangled steamships and trains crisscrossed oceans and continents, carrying the goods produced in the factories. The expansion of trade allowed diseases to spread more easily. The transportation boom overwhelmed existing quarantine procedures. Nations responded

THE FATHER OF MODERN PUBLIC HEALTH

English social reformer Edwin Chadwick (1800–1890) helped bring about his country's first public health laws. Trained as a lawyer, Chadwick began to work in 1832 on a commission making revisions to the Poor Laws, which governed social services provided to England's poor. In this role, Chadwick championed ideas that were radical for his time. He argued that the government could improve public health by improving living conditions in poor neighborhoods. As a result of the Industrial Revolution, tens of thousands of people had flocked to England's cities, particularly London, in search of factory jobs. Crowded, filthy, and disease-ridden slums grew.

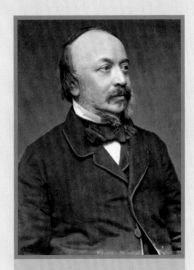

English politician and social reformer Sir Edwin Chadwick, who dedicated his career to sanitary reform and public health in Great Britain.

In an 1842 report, Chadwick wrote that diseases in poor neighborhoods were a threat to all Britons. He asserted that Britain's poor had the right to decent living conditions. Five years by strengthening their quarantine laws. These tougher laws, however, angered powerful merchants. Longer quarantine periods created longer delays at ports, harming businesses. Doctors and government officials noted that the new quarantine laws had little effect on the spread of diseases.

later, Chadwick headed a commission that studied sanitary conditions in London. The commission's report advocated separating the city's sewage system from its water drainage system.

In 1848, a cholera epidemic struck England, killing as many as 10,000 people in London. The government took action, adopting many of Chadwick's recommendations. Parliament enacted groundbreaking sanitary and public health laws known as the Public Health Act of 1848. This act would provide the foundation for modern public health services.

The Public Health Act set up a government bureau to provide health education, vaccination programs to control diseases, and agencies to test and inspect water supplies, foods, and drugs. It also started government sanitation projects that supplied clean water and introduced effective trash and sewage removal in neighborhoods rich and poor. (At the time, many people, including Chadwick, thought that unpleasant odors from sewage and trash could cause disease.)

The act also established a Board of Health. Chadwick was appointed as a commissioner. His career in public health did not last long, however. Chadwick's reforms met opposition from several sources. Political foes did not want to fund his public work projects. Engineers ridiculed his plans for sewers. Doctors argued that only doctors should serve on the Board of Health. Chadwick was pressured to resign from the board in 1854.

To satisfy the demand for more raw materials for their factories, European businesses began to import these products from colonies in Africa, Asia, and the Americas. The many ships returning from ports on these continents increased the risk of new diseases. Cholera, a disease previously unknown in Europe, struck the continent in 1831. The epidemic killed tens of thousands of people. Another cholera epidemic ravaged Europe in 1848.

Some countries and cities responded to the rise in epidemics by establishing national sanitary organizations. The first sanitary organization—the Sanitary, Medicine, and Quarantine Board of Alexandria, Egypt—was founded in the 1830s. Rather than relying on quarantines to protect people from diseases being introduced from abroad, these sanitary organizations focused on improving the living conditions within their own countries.

In response to the devastating cholera epidemic of 1848, doctors from many countries felt that action needed to be taken on an international scale. They organized the first International Sanitary Conference in 1851. Meeting in Paris, France, delegates discussed quarantine policies and other ways to prevent the spread of cholera. Because medical researchers at the time had discovered very little about cholera (as well as other diseases), the conference never achieved its goal of preventing the spread of the deadly disease.

Over the next century, countries increased their cooperation on health issues. Individual nations and new international organizations addressed the most serious threats to public health. International sanitary conferences were held about every five years. The delegates to these conferences developed and adopted guidelines that helped countries to negotiate treaties to control infectious diseases. These agreements focused mainly on controlling the spread of plague, cholera, yellow fever, and other diseases from Europe's colonial territories in Asia, Africa, and the Americas.

EARLY TWENTIETH-CENTURY ORGANIZATIONS

Remarkable new scientific discoveries in the late nineteenth and early twentieth centuries led to more effective international public health rules and policies. By 1900, scientists had developed an explanation for the cause of some diseases. It became known as germ theory. According to this theory, microbes can invade the body and cause some diseases and infections. Microbes are microorganisms that are too small to be seen except through a microscope. The discoveries of French chemist Louis Pasteur, English surgeon Joseph Lister, and German doctor Robert Koch became the major components of germ theory. Recognizing the potential of germ theory to identify the microbes that cause disease, Pasteur predicted, "It is in the power of man to make parasitic maladies disappear from the face of the earth."[5]

These scientific and medical discoveries revolutionized sanitary and public health policies. Government officials began to adopt public health measures to prevent the spread of disease. These measures included improving water supplies and sewage systems and vaccinating healthy people. New public health laws and procedures reduced the spread of diseases in communities and between nations. The existing international treaties and quarantine policies, however, proved less effective. Changing treaties and quarantine laws took a lot of time. It was difficult to keep them up to date with the latest scientific knowledge about infectious diseases. Doctors and government officials around the world began to encourage the development of new ways to combat infectious diseases.

The world's first global health organization was founded in 1902 by countries in North and South America. The International Sanitary Bureau collected regional data on the frequency, cause, and distribution of diseases in the Americas. It exchanged this epidemiological information with other health organizations. The association's name was later changed to the Pan American Health Organization. The organization would play an active role in the extensive campaign to eradicate yellow fever in the Americas.

At the eleventh International Sanitary Conference in 1903, delegates from around the world agreed that a permanent international health organization should be created. It could coordinate quarantine measures worldwide and gather and publish epidemiological data and information. Four years later, nine European countries, plus Egypt, Brazil, and the United States signed the Rome Agreement, which created the Office International d'Hygiène Publique (OIHP). (In English, the organization's name was the International Office of Public Hygiene.) OIHP's mission was to distribute to member states information on general public health, particularly on infectious diseases and how to combat them. Financed by its member nations, OIHP had its headquarters in Paris. Within seven years, membership grew to 60 nations. During its early years, the organization focused on overseeing and improving international quarantine policies. OIHP adopted policies that required nations to notify it of any outbreak of major infectious diseases, such as cholera, plague, or yellow fever.

Several pandemics (widespread epidemics) swept through Europe at the end of World War I (1914–1918) and in the following years. The influenza wave of 1918–1919 killed an estimated 15 million to 20 million people. Influenza was not the only disease that ravaged the continent. In 1919, nearly 2 million cases of typhus were reported in Poland and the Soviet Union. OIHP did not have the resources to respond effectively to such large epidemics.

In 1919, 44 nations signed an agreement to establish the League of Nations. This new organization was the first international effort to create a cooperative system to settle disputes between countries. The hope was that diplomacy would help nations avoid future wars. Among its early activities, the league set up its own international health organization. The mission of the Health Organization of the League of Nations would extend beyond OIHP's existing role. The League of Nations gave its agency authority to take a more active role in dealing with infectious diseases.

With the creation of this new organization, OIHP made plans to cease operations in 1920 and transfer its responsibilities to the Health Organization of the League of Nations. OIHP, however, did not close down. The U.S. Senate refused to approve the treaty that would have made the United States a member of the League of Nations. Along with two other nations, the United States kept OIHP operating. It continued to work independently of the League of Nation's health organization. A rivalry between the two organizations grew.

The Health Organization of the League of Nations focused its early work on responding to and preventing epidemics. For example, it worked with the Soviet Union to provide education on typhus. Its Malaria Commission pursued a new approach to controlling that infectious disease. The commission abandoned efforts to develop procedures to prevent the spread of malaria from country to country. Instead, it studied the disease in the regions where it was widespread and advised countries on ways to control the disease locally. The organization's Cancer Commission provided doctors and health officials in member countries with the latest research on various types of cancer.

As an international organization, the League of Nations proved to be weak and ineffective. It failed in its primary mission: containing conflict between nations. A new world war broke out in 1939, eventually involving most of the countries in the world. World War II halted the operations of both the Health Organization of the League of Nations and OIHP.

After the war, many countries lay in ruin. The war had killed about 50 million people worldwide. The world's nations wanted to ensure that such a catastrophic war would never occur again. They banded together to create a much stronger international organization than the League of Nations. Its primary mission would be to maintain peace between countries. Representatives

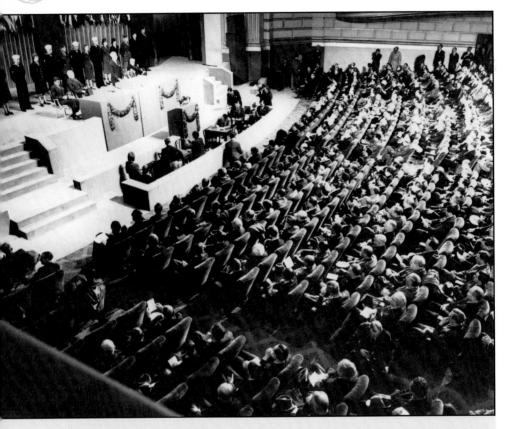

Representatives from 50 countries (later 51) convened in San Francisco to draw up the United Nations Charter on April 25, 1945. One of the issues they discussed was the establishment of a global health organization. April 7, 2008, marked the sixtieth anniversary of the World Health Organization.

from the world's nations met in San Francisco in April 1945. They drafted a treaty known as the United Nations Charter. Originally signed by 51 nations, the charter created the United Nations. (Almost every country has now signed the charter.) The UN's mission is to help nations work together on issues of world peace, international law and security, human rights, and economic and social development.

The idea for a UN specialized agency for health was proposed at a 1946 meeting of the UN's Economic and Social

Council. The council agreed to organize an international health conference. In June 1946, delegates from all 51 UN member states, along with delegates from 13 nonmember countries, met in New York City. During the monthlong conference, the delegates agreed on a constitution for a new international health organization.

The World Health Organization formally came into existence in September 1948, when the twenty-sixth UN member state ratified WHO's constitution. It took control of the work of the Health Organization of the League of Nations and OIHP. Both organizations were dissolved. Although the two groups had never worked together, they had provided a foundation for expanding cooperation among countries to improve global public health. The world's other major international health organization, the Pan American Health Organization, joined WHO. It became the regional office for the Americas.

In its early years, WHO focused on rebuilding health services in war-torn countries. It targeted several key diseases, particularly malaria, tuberculosis, and sexually transmitted diseases like syphilis. It also worked hard to improve nutrition, mother-and-child health, and sanitation standards.

In 1951, WHO produced a new set of international rules to control infectious disease. The International Sanitary Regulations established standardized procedures for countries to notify WHO of any major disease outbreaks and for handling infected international travelers and cargo. Updated in 1969 and expanded in 1973 and 1981, these rules are now known as the International Health Regulations.

During the 1950s, WHO membership grew rapidly. Former European colonies in Africa, Asia, and Latin America gained their independence and joined the organization. With more members, WHO's budget also grew. It was able to expand existing programs and projects and to create new ones.

The growth of WHO, however, created a rift among its member nations. Many of WHO's newer members were poor, less-developed countries. During the 1960s and 1970s, they voiced their desire for the organization to provide different types of health services. Most of the programs that WHO had adopted in the past mirrored the health-care models of rich, developed countries. WHO concentrated its efforts on helping to build hospitals in large cities and providing health services to patients suffering from diseases. This approach usually required highly trained medical staff and expensive medical technology. The model worked well in rich countries. It was not a good fit, however, for most poor, developing countries. They had few well-trained doctors and could not afford the most up-to-date medical technology. Instead, these countries wanted WHO to help them develop community-based health-care systems that were affordable.

During the 1970s, under the leadership of Director-General Halfdan Mahler, WHO changed its approach. The organization began to focus on a new health-care model, known as primary health care. The goal of primary health care was to provide medical services appropriate to a country's needs, wealth, and culture. These community-based systems would use practical, medically sound, and socially acceptable methods. They would use technologies that a community and a country could afford.

To implement primary health-care systems in poor countries, WHO provided education on common local health problems and methods to prevent and control diseases. The organization focused on programs to provide an adequate supply of food and safe water, basic sanitation methods, proper nutrition, and mother-and-child health care. It also created programs that provided essential drugs and vaccinations against major infectious diseases.

WHO's primary health-care programs helped build hundreds of rural health centers. Thousands of community health workers were trained worldwide. The movement away from high-tech, urban hospitals expanded the reach of public health in developing countries. These new low-tech, locally appropriate, community-based approaches helped improve the health of many more people.

During the 1980s, WHO faced many difficult challenges. Disagreeing with the direction of the UN, the United States began to withhold funds from the UN and its agencies, including WHO. Without funding from the UN's richest member state, WHO suffered a financial shortfall. Having less money in its budget had a major impact on many programs.

Other organizations also began to enter the field of international health care during the decade. Another UN specialized agency, the World Bank, began to work in the health field. Founded in 1944, the World Bank was created to provide loans and other grants to developing countries. It became well known for its successes in helping developing countries improve their government services, develop their financial sectors, and build their infrastructures. Its loans helped to build roads, bridges, and dams throughout the developing world. In the 1980s, the World Bank began to provide loans to developing countries to build up their health programs. By 1990, it became the largest source of money for health-care programs in the world. The World Bank began to hire public health professionals and started its own health programs. Other UN organizations, such as UNICEF and the UN High Commission on Refugees, also developed their own health programs. The European Union and various nongovernmental agencies, such as the Red Cross, also created health programs. These new competitors and their health programs made WHO's role in international public health less clear.

Still, WHO continued to combat new challenges. WHO's Global Program on AIDS was one of its major successes in the 1980s. In 1987, the UN General Assembly recognized HIV/AIDS as a "worldwide emergency" and called on WHO to play the "essential directing and coordinating role" within the UN in fighting HIV/AIDS.[6] WHO received funding from many sources, enabling it to hire staff to develop national HIV/AIDS strategies for more than 170 countries.

During the 1990s, WHO began to refashion itself. While the World Bank's greatest advantage was its tremendous economic influence, it recognized that WHO had considerable expertise in health and medicine. In 1998, Gro Harlem Brundtland, a physician and former prime minister of Norway, became WHO's director-general. She wanted to turn WHO into an organization that influenced others on the global scene. She began to strengthen WHO's financial position and organized global partnerships that brought together private donors, governments, and international agencies.

In 2008, WHO celebrated its sixtieth anniversary. WHO remains the foremost source of scientific and technical knowledge in international public health. It shares the information it gathers with its member nations and other international organizations through meetings, publications, and cooperative programs. WHO has also taken on the role of the world's health conscience. It advocates principles of equality in health care for all of the world's people.

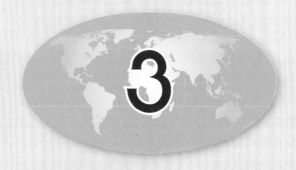

WHO at Work

THE WORLD HEALTH ORGANIZATION HAS THREE MAJOR branches: the World Health Assembly (WHA), the Executive Board, and the Secretariat. These three groups determine WHO's policies and carry out its programs in order to fulfill the organization's mission to provide leadership on global health issues.

WORLD HEALTH ASSEMBLY

The World Health Assembly is the legislative and policy branch of WHO. Since 1948, the assembly has met each year, usually in May, for two weeks at WHO's headquarters in Geneva, Switzerland. The assembly consists of representatives from all 193 member states. Each nation has one vote but may send up to three representatives to the annual conference.

Representatives of other international and nongovernmental organizations also attend the sessions as observers.

The assembly's representatives vote on a wide range of resolutions, from creating public health policies and adopting international health regulations to approving the organization's budget. The goal is for representatives to reach a consensus on each resolution presented to them. The assembly approves a resolution if it receives two-thirds of the total vote. A president, who is selected by the assembly, chairs the annual conference. Representatives express their views on resolutions and

 A WHO RESOLUTION

The sixty-first session of the World Health Assembly adopted a resolution to develop a global plan to reduce the harmful use of alcohol. In many countries, the use of alcohol causes a substantial health, social, and economic burden. In its resolution, the assembly urged member states "to collaborate with the Secretariat in developing a draft global strategy on harmful use of alcohol based on all evidence and best strategies."* It also requested the WHO director-general "to ensure that the draft global strategy will include a set of proposed measures recommended for states to implement at the national level, taking into account the national circumstances of each country."** The director-general was also instructed "to collaborate and consult with member states as well as consult with intergovernmental organizations, health professionals, nongovernmental organizations, and economic operators on ways they could contribute to reducing harmful use of alcohol."*** The assembly asked the director-general to submit a draft of the WHO global strategy to reduce harmful use of alcohol to the 63rd World Health Assembly, via the Executive Board.

encourage all nations to follow WHO directives. The assembly also supervises and evaluates the work of the Executive Board and the Secretariat.

More than 2,700 participants from 190 nations met at the 61st World Health Assembly held in 2008. They took action against new threats to global public health. In 2008, the assembly endorsed a major resolution to promote pharmaceutical research and development. It adopted new approaches to improve and make more affordable the development of drugs to prevent and treat diseases that have a major impact on developing countries.

The World Health Assembly was particularly concerned about alcohol use by teens. Alcohol is the number one drug of choice for young people, and its use has become a major cause of teen injuries (particularly from traffic accidents), violence and crime involving teens (especially domestic violence, assaults, rapes, and vandalism), and premature teen deaths (drownings, fires, suicides, and homicides). Alcohol use also has a negative effect on school attendance and performance. A 2007 study provided evidence that young people around the world are starting to drink at an earlier age. Drinking by young people can cause physical harm to the brain, which continues to mature until age 25.

* Sixty-First World Health Assembly. Agenda item 11.10, WHA61.4., May 24, 2008, "Strategies to Reduce the Harmful Use of Alcohol." Available online at *http://www.who.int/nmh/WHA%2061.4.pdf.*

** Ibid.

*** Ibid.

WHO Headquarters Structure (Excluding Partnerships Secretariats)

World Health Assembly

Executive Board

Secretariat

Director-General
Deputy Director-General
Executive Director
Advisers
Governing Bodies
Internal Oversight Services
Legal Counsel

Communications
Ombudsmen
Public Health, Innovation,
   and Intellectual Property
Secretariat to the Framework
   Convention on Tobacco Control

Family and Community Health

Ageing and Life Course
Child and Adolescent Health and Development
Gender, Women, and Health
Immunization, Vaccines, and Biologicals
Making Pregnancy Safer
Reproductive Health and Research

General Management

Finance
Global Learning and Performance Management
Global Service Center
Human Resources Management
Information Technology and
   Telecommunications
Operational Support and Services
Planning, Resource Coordination,
   and Performance Monitoring

Health Action in Crises

Emergency Preparedness and Capacity Building
Emergency Response and Operations
Recovery and Transition Programs
Special Assignments
WHO Mediterranean Center for
   Vulnerability Reduction, Tunis

**Health Security and Environment and the
Representative of the Director-General
for Polio Eradication**

Epidemic and Pandemic Alert and Response
Food Safety, Zoonoses, and Foodborne Diseases
Polio Eradication Initiative
Protection of the Human Environment

Health Systems and Services

Essential Health Technologies
Essential Medicines and Pharmeceutical Policies
Health System Governance and Service Delivery
Health System Financing
Human Resources for Health

**HIV/AIDS, TB, Malaria and
Neglected Tropical Diseases**

Control of Neglected Tropical Diseases
Global Malaria Program
HIV/AIDS
Stop TB

Information, Evidence and Research

Ethics, Equity, Trade and Human Rights
Knowledge Management and Sharing
Measurement and Health Information Systems
Research Policy and Cooperation
Special Program for Research and
   Training in Tropical Diseases

**Noncommunicable Diseases
and Mental Health**

Chronic Diseases and Health Promotion
Mental Health and Substance Abuse
Nutrition for Health and Development
Tobacco Free Initiative
Violence and Injury Prevention and Disability
WHO Center for Health Development, Kobe

Partnerships and United Nations Reform
Partnerships and United Nations
Country Focus

WHO Offices at the:
African Union and the Economic Commission
   for Africa, Addis Ababa
European Union, Brussels
United Nations, New York

© Infobase Publishing

The assembly also approved a six-year plan to reduce the effects of chronic diseases, such as cardiovascular diseases, diabetes, and cancers. These diseases cause about 60 percent of all deaths worldwide. The assembly adopted another resolution that urged member states to address the impact of climate change on health. It also directed the Secretariat to help countries in reaching a higher percentage of immunization and to encourage the development of new vaccines. Although vaccines prevent as many as 3 million deaths a year, the assembly noted that WHO vaccination programs should be expanded.

THE EXECUTIVE BOARD

WHO's Executive Board is responsible for making sure that resolutions passed by the World Health Assembly are carried out. Six regional committees nominate member nations to serve on the board. Each country that is elected to join the Executive Board then selects a qualified health expert to serve as a board member. Members of the Executive Board customarily do not act as representatives of their respective governments. Instead, they are counted on to make their decisions in the best interests of international public health.

The 34 board members serve three-year terms. Each year, about one-third of the Executive Board members are replaced. The Executive Board usually includes members from at least three of the five permanent members of the United Nations Security Council. Those countries are China, France, Russia, the United Kingdom, and the United States.

The Executive Board meets twice a year. In January, board members meet to prepare for the annual World Health Assembly

(Opposite page) The mission of WHO is "the attainment by all peoples of the highest possible level of health." All UN members are eligible to join WHO. Currently there are 193 member states. The World Health Assembly is the supreme decision-making body of WHO and is composed of health ministers from member states.

conference held in May. They draft agendas, resolutions, and budget proposals for assembly representatives to consider. After the conference, the Executive Board meets to take care of administrative tasks. Its duties also include drafting the WHO's six-year strategic plan, known as the General Program of Work. The board also advises the Secretariat on constitutional or organizational issues. The Executive Board has the power to take emergency measures whenever necessary.

THE SECRETARIAT

The Secretariat is responsible for carrying out WHO's day-to-day operations. It includes the director-general, doctors, public health professionals, and administrative workers. The Secretariat has three main divisions: headquarters, regional offices, and country offices. About one-third of WHO employees work in each of these divisions. The WHO is more decentralized than most of the other 13 UN specialized agencies. More than 8,000 people work for WHO. They come from many countries and serve for a set period of time.

The Director-General

The director-general is the executive head of WHO. She or he serves as the organization's top public health officer and as its chief administrative officer. The director-general's responsibilities include appointing WHO staff, preparing annual financial statements, and representing WHO in UN meetings and other events.

An amendment to WHO's constitution spells out the necessary qualifications for a director-general. These include a strong background in public health, the ability to manage a large organization, and an understanding of cultural, social, and political differences between nations. Member states can recommend qualified applicants for the director-general post. From these many candidates, the Executive Board chooses a

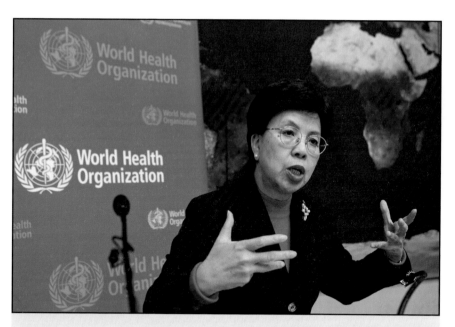

Margaret Chan was elected director-general of WHO by the Executive Board on November 8, 2006. Chan was selected over 12 other candidates to become leader of the organization due to her successful handling of the 1997 avian flu outbreak and the 2003 SARS outbreak in Hong Kong. During that time she was the first female head of Hong Kong's Department of Health.

nominee. The World Health Assembly then votes to approve the nomination. Once approved, the director-general serves a five-year term.

The director-general and many other employees work in WHO's headquarters in Geneva, Switzerland. In 1948, WHO took charge of the offices of the former Health Organization of the League of Nations. The organization moved its headquarters into its own new building in 1968. Besides its many offices, WHO's headquarters has conference halls, an extensive medical and public health library, and facilities for printing and distributing its many publications.

Regional Offices

Regional offices are responsible for carrying out the decisions of the World Health Assembly and the Executive Board within their respective regions. The director-general oversees the work of the regional offices. The six regional offices are:

1. Regional Office for Africa, headquartered in Brazzaville, Congo.
2. Regional Office for the Americas, headquartered in Washington, D.C.
3. Regional Office for the Eastern Mediterranean, headquartered in Cairo, Egypt.
4. Regional Office for Europe, headquartered in Copenhagen, Denmark.
5. Regional Office for Southeast Asia, headquartered in New Delhi, India.
6. Regional Office for the Western Pacific, headquartered in Manila, Philippines.

The regional offices allow WHO to build good relationships and maintain effective contact with national governments. This is a key function because these governments are responsible for implementing many of WHO's programs and initiatives. These offices also monitor regional health issues.

Each regional office differs in structure and personnel, depending on the specific needs of the region. Each region has a committee made up of representatives from its member states. Each committee nominates a director for its region; the Executive Board appoints the director.

The regional director serves as both the public health and the administrative head of the regional office. Because of the decentralized nature of WHO, regional directors play a major role in the organization. They are responsible for planning and managing programs. They also oversee their region's budget and appoint WHO representatives to country offices in their region.

Country Offices

Country offices are located within each member state. They are often based in the host country's national health department. Professional staff members, temporary technical advisers and consultants, and support staff work in country offices. A WHO representative heads each country office. The representative keeps the regional director informed of any special health problems in the country.

The main function of country offices is to develop and manage programs at the country level. They work with the country's national health department to implement a wide variety of WHO programs and policies. For example, WHO's Bangladesh office worked with that country's Ministry of Health and Family Welfare to implement programs that provide safe drinking water. According to some estimates, high levels of arsenic in the water supplies in some areas of Bangladesh cause about 200,000 deaths a year. Prolonged consumption of high levels of arsenic can lead to cancers, heart diseases, diabetes, and other serious health problems. Other examples of WHO country programs are the WHO Collaborating Center on Ultraviolet Radiation and Its Health Effects in Bolivia and the WHO Health System Review in Estonia.

Norwegian doctor Eigil Sörensen is WHO's country representative in Papua New Guinea. "I enjoy contributing to tackling major public health problems in countries," Sörensen observed. "Working as WHO representative is a challenge. It requires the use of personal and technical skills and knowledge, and provides many opportunities to influence important health programs. I enjoy finding the right balance between working with the country while also being an independent observer and advocate for people's health needs."[7]

WHO IN ACTION

The public health leaders who founded WHO wanted the organization to operate in almost every field of global health.

WHO's constitution provides a broad framework for the organization to meet its objective to attain the highest level of health for the world's people. Article 2 of the constitution names 22 specific functions for the organization to pursue. The most basic function is to adopt resolutions, make agreements, and establish regulations to improve global health. These activities provide the foundation for WHO's wide variety of programs, publications, and partnerships.

Health Programs

Much of WHO's work is focused on health programs and projects. The organization is perhaps best known for its efforts to eradicate diseases and control outbreaks of infectious diseases. When a country asks for help, WHO provides appropriate technical assistance, including medical services and training as well as emergency aid.

WHO provides direct assistance to governments to respond to specific health needs or to strengthen national or local health systems. Low- and middle-income countries receive most of this type of assistance. In providing services, WHO follows the principle that every nation's sovereignty (self-rule) should be respected. Each country has the right to develop its own health system and services in a way that its government finds most sensible and appropriate to its needs.

WHO operates a wide variety of health programs and projects. A few programs and projects that demonstrate WHO's range and reach are:

- Diabetes Program, which seeks to prevent diabetes, help diabetics, and raise awareness of the disease.
- Department of Control of Neglected Tropical Diseases, which seeks to eliminates yaws, Chagas' disease, leprosy, schistosomiasis, and other tropical diseases. In 2004, the department announced that its efforts had

helped eliminate yaws—a disease that primarily affects the skin, bones, and cartilage—in India.

- Department of Ethics, Trade, Human Rights, and Health Law, which helps ensure that all WHO programs and policies incorporate the principles of dignity, justice, and security.
- Global Database on Child Growth and Malnutrition, which compiles data from nutritional surveys conducted around the world since 1960.
- Health Workforce, which provides education, training, and other services to improve the distribution and performance of health workers.
- Global Advisory Committee on Vaccine Safety, which monitors and responds to vaccine-safety issues of worldwide importance.

WHO also provides emergency assistance to nations in need. Epidemics, wars and political unrest, and natural disasters like earthquakes, floods, and hurricanes often strike without warning. Major health emergencies can occur anywhere in the world. In May 2008, for example, WHO responded to a powerful earthquake that struck China. Centered in Sichuan Province, the earthquake affected more than 350 million people in eight provinces. It damaged or destroyed more than 16 million buildings. Five million people were displaced. More than 65,000 people were killed, and about 100,000 were hospitalized with injuries. WHO worked with the UN's Disaster Management Team and China's Ministry of Health to identify priority needs and obtain supplies. Once the short-term health services were provided, WHO's Communicable Disease Working Group focused on lessening the risk factors for cholera, measles, pneumonia, and other communicable diseases. This work involved providing safe food, clean water, and adequate shelter.

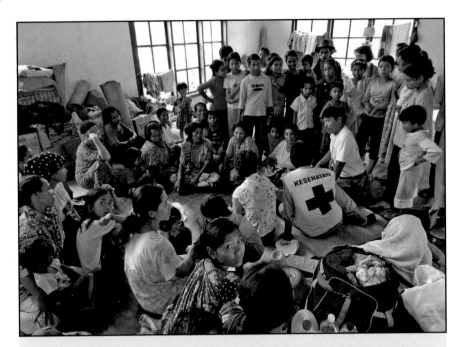

After a series of devastating tsunami in southern Asia killed more than 225,000 people in 11 countries, WHO partnered with several organizations to provide emergency assistance. WHO reported that, in addition to the grief felt from the loss of loved ones, homes, livelihood, and entire community networks, there was also a shortage of mental health workers to offer counseling. In response, WHO and its partners trained community-based workers to incorporate a culturally appropriate approach for each region.

Research and Health Information

Two key WHO functions are promoting and conducting research and collecting health statistics and epidemiological information. WHO publishes health information in a variety of publications. Launched in 1995, *World Health Report* is WHO's most important publication. It reports on the state of human health worldwide, providing up-to-date statistical data on major health issues and the health status of specific population centers. This data gives countries, donor agencies, international organizations, and other users the latest medical and public health information they need to make policy and funding decisions. The report also provides students, health-care professionals, and others with critical information on international health issues.

World Health Report focuses on a specific theme each year. The 2008 *World Health Report*, for example, proposed ways to improve primary health-care systems. Subtitled *Working Together for Health*, it identified four goals:

1. Achieving universal access to primary care.
2. Restructuring health-care services to meet patients' needs and expectations.
3. Adopting better national health-care policies to attain healthier communities.
4. Encouraging more effective government participation.

Other WHO publications include *World Health Statistics Annual* and *World Health Statistics Quarterly, International Lists of Causes of Death, International Nomenclature of Diseases,* and *International Health Regulations.*

WHO also enacts international rules that establish standards and naming conventions for foods, pharmaceuticals, and similar products. To foster the global exchange of health information and ideas, WHO also promotes cooperation among scientists and public health experts.

Accomplishing Its Mission

Each year, the World Health Assembly adopts a General Program of Work report, which outlines the organization's primary activities for the next six years. The report provides a broad framework for WHO's policies. All activities noted in the report relate to WHO's core functions:

- Providing leadership on issues critical to global public health.
- Encouraging the creation and distribution of valuable medical and public-health knowledge.
- Setting norms and standards for public health.
- Creating health-care policy options that are based on scientific evidence and ethical considerations.
- Providing technical support and developing sustainable programs.
- Monitoring global public health and assessing trends.

To carry out its mission, WHO often partners with other international organizations in joint projects. For example, the Roll Back Malaria Partnership is a coordinated effort to reduce cases of malaria worldwide. The United Nations Development Program, UNICEF, the World Bank, and WHO launched the partnership in 1998. Since its founding, the partnership has grown, with new members including nongovernmental organizations, private corporations, and countries where malaria is endemic. World Blood Donor Day, another partnership program, promotes blood donation around the globe. WHO cosponsors the event with the International Federation of Blood Donor Organizations, the International Society of Blood Transfusion, and the International Federation of Red Cross and Red Crescent Societies.

ORGANIZATIONAL CHALLENGES

WHO faces two major organizational challenges: overcoming the strained relations between member nations and achieving its mission despite a limited budget. Both of these challenges have proven difficult to solve in the past. They require diplomacy, negotiation, and the development of new approaches to funding the organization.

Since the 1960s, international politics and an increased sense of regionalism have led to conflicts at the World Health

Assembly. (Regionalism is a sense of shared identity and goals expressed by countries in a specific geographical area.) These conflicts have made it more difficult for the Secretariat to carry out WHO programs. The most serious ongoing rift among WHO members is between rich and poor members. Governments of poor nations disagree with the governments of wealthier nations on what WHO's mission should be. Most poor- and middle-income nations want the organization to focus its resources on helping their governments combat specific diseases and strengthen national primary health-care systems. Wealthier countries see a narrower mission for WHO. They want the organization to concentrate its efforts on managing disease programs, providing technical expertise, and gathering and distributing international public health information. This tension has hindered the effectiveness of WHO.

Money to operate WHO comes from two sources: regular budget funds and extra-budgetary funds. Regular budget funds come from the contributions charged to each member state. Nations do not all make the same contribution. Each nation's payment is based on its ability to pay, which is determined by its wealth and population. Wealthy countries—including the United States, Germany, and Japan—make larger contributions to WHO than poorer countries like Somalia, Nicaragua, and Cambodia.

Extra-budgetary funds come from donations to the organization. Member states often provide funds in addition to their regular contributions. Other UN organizations, private organizations, and individuals also donate money to WHO. Some of these donations are given for a specific program or use. For example, the United States made large donations to WHO's malaria- and smallpox-eradication programs. When a donation comes with attached conditions—for example, it must be spent on mother-and-child health—the Executive Board must review the donation. If the board approves of the conditions, WHO can accept the donation. In the 1990s, extra-budgetary funding surpassed regular budget funding for the first time. This change occurred as WHO shifted its focus from disease programs to primary health programs. The future success of WHO's programs will depend on the commitment of its member nations and access to adequate financial resources.

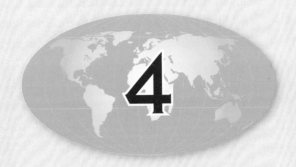

The UN Millennium Development Goals

In 2000, REPRESENTATIVES FROM 189 NATIONS MET AT THE United Nations' Millennium Summit. They adopted a ground-breaking initiative called the Millennium Declaration. They agreed that their common goal was to "free our fellow men, women, and children from the abject and dehumanizing conditions of extreme poverty, to which more than a billion of them are currently subjected."[8] One hundred and forty-seven nations signed the declaration. For the first time in history, most of the world's governments committed themselves to improving the lives of people worldwide by addressing poverty and poor health. Low-income countries pledged to improve their health policies and governance. They also agreed to increase their accountability to their citizens. Wealthy countries promised to provide the resources needed.

In the Millennium Declaration, nations agreed to a set of eight goals. The fulfillment of these goals would end extreme poverty by 2015. To ensure that governments would work toward reaching the goals, each nation agreed to have the progress of its development activities monitored. In addition, major international financial institutions—such as the World Bank, the International Monetary Fund, and the World Trade Organization—agreed to be accountable for achieving the goals. As one of the United Nations' specialized agencies, WHO also promised its support and agreed to help achieve the goals of the Millennium Declaration.

MILLENNIUM DEVELOPMENT GOALS

To meet the world's main development challenges, the Millennium Declaration stressed a wide range of actions and targets. The declaration identified eight specific goals to be achieved by 2015. These became known as the Millennium Development Goals. They are:

Goal 1   Eradicate extreme poverty and hunger.
Goal 2   Achieve universal primary education.
Goal 3   Promote gender equality and empower women.
Goal 4   Reduce child mortality.
Goal 5   Improve maternal health.
Goal 6   Combat HIV/AIDS, malaria, and other diseases.
Goal 7   Ensure environmental sustainability.
Goal 8   Build a global partnership for development.

To achieve these goals, the UN also adopted various targets for each one. Meeting these targets would show how much progress had been made toward the goals.

The adoption of the millennium goals had a profound impact on the work of WHO. Health issues are a major part of the goals. Three of them deal directly with health: reducing child mortality, improving maternal health, and combating

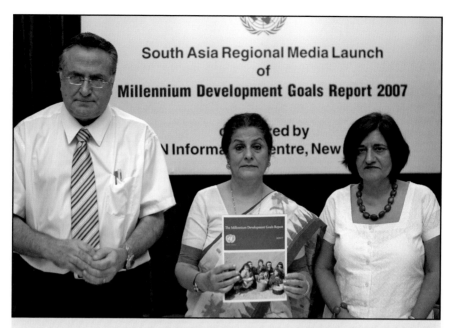

In July 2007, the WHO regional office in India released the Millennium Development Goals Report 2007, an annual statistical survey produced at the request of the UN General Assembly that outlines their region's global and regional progress toward the Millennium Goals. This report came at the midpoint of a 15-year effort to implement a set of eight key development objectives that world leaders pledged to achieve by 2015.

HIV/AIDS, malaria, and other diseases. Health is also a component of the other five goals.

WHO is strengthening its presence within member nations to help those countries meet their goals, and it is working with other UN organizations to identify indicators for each health-related goal. WHO monitors and tracks progress within countries, helping to identify programs and methods that make a measurable improvement in public health. This chapter examines WHO's role in achieving goals 4 and 5 and its less central role in achieving goals 1, 2, 3, 7, and 8. The next chapter focuses on the organization's major role in achieving Goal 6, combating HIV/AIDS, malaria, and other diseases.

REDUCING CHILD MORTALITY

Child-mortality statistics demonstrate the importance of Goal 4—reducing the number of child deaths. Nearly 10 million children under the age of five die each year. About 4 million infants each year die within the first 28 days of life. Nearly 99 percent of childhood deaths occur in low- and middle-income countries, mostly in sub-Saharan Africa and South Asia.

Studies have shown that many of these deaths would be preventable if children had access to community-based health services. Six major diseases or factors cause about 90 percent of all deaths of children under the age of six. They are diarrhea, HIV/AIDS, malaria, measles, neonatal causes (such as infection, premature delivery, and lack of oxygen at birth), and pneumonia. Malnutrition and the lack of safe water and sanitation contribute to about half of all these children's deaths.

One target of Goal 4 is to reduce by two-thirds the mortality rate of children under the age of five. In 1990, 93 children out of every 1,000 born died before reaching age five. The goal's target is to reduce that number to 31 out of every 1,000 by 2015. (By comparison, industrialized countries have an average rate of six deaths by age five for every 1,000 children.)

In meeting this goal, WHO is working with other international agencies and national health departments to reduce the rate of child deaths. It provides technical advice (including information on combating specific diseases) and policy support (such as training for health-care workers). To help doctors, researchers, and public health officials better understand child mortality, WHO collects data on the under-five mortality rate, the infant mortality rate, and the proportion of one-year-old children who have been immunized against measles.

Working with UNICEF, WHO has developed the Global Immunization Vision and Strategy. This strategy aims to immunize more people, with a focus on children, throughout the world. Its main goal is, by 2015, to reduce illness and death due to vaccine-preventable diseases by at least two-thirds of the

2000 level. The program also seeks to introduce new vaccines, ensure access to good-quality vaccines, and monitor vaccination programs. WHO's immunization efforts have helped save the lives of many children. Serigne Dame Leye, chief of Nguoye Diaraf village in the West African nation of Senegal, praised a WHO immunization program, saying, "We used to bury two or three children every week during measles epidemics. This does not happen anymore."[9] In 2008, WHO worked with UNICEF to help the Ivory Coast conduct a nationwide measles vaccination campaign. More than 3 million children age nine months to five years received a vaccination.

The estimated price tag for immunization activities for 2006–2015 is $35 billion. One-third of this amount will be allocated to buying vaccines. The remaining two-thirds will be spent on creating immunization delivery systems. WHO and UNICEF estimate that the Global Immunization Vision and Strategy's vaccination program will save 10 million lives.

WHO's Children's Environmental Health program works to support safe, healthy, and clean environments for young people. Of the world's 6.7 billion people, 1.8 billion are age 14 or younger. Child survival and development depend on having a safe, healthy, and clean environment. Environmental factors, such as the presence of irrigation water, cause about 90 percent of malaria cases worldwide. (Infected mosquitoes transmit malaria to humans by carrying malaria protozoa from person to person. They reproduce by laying their eggs in stagnant water.) About 800,000 children under the age of five die from malaria each year. Eighty percent to 90 percent of diarrhea deaths worldwide are related to contaminated water, inadequate sanitation, and other environmental conditions. Diarrheal diseases claim the lives of about 1.7 million children every year. Environmental conditions, such as smoke from cooking fires, are a factor in as many as 60 percent of acute respiratory infections. Such infections annually kill an estimated 2 million children under the age of five.

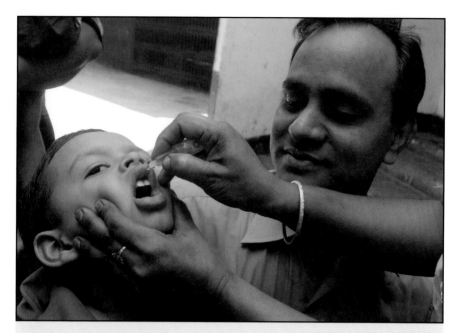

Today, immunizations save more than 3 million lives. Still, 15 million people die each year from preventable diseases due to lack of access to basic health care and immunizations. In response, WHO has pledged to help developing countries to immunize all children and eligible adults. It has had several successes in the Western Pacific region within the last decade, including achieving polio-free status and the reduction of measles deaths by 95 percent.

The Children's Environmental Health program educates and trains health-care providers on how to diagnose, manage, and prevent children's diseases linked to environmental risk factors. It promotes research into children's environmental health. This research helps transfer medical knowledge from wealthy countries to middle- and low-income countries. It also helps developing countries build health-care systems to deal with environmental risk factors. Two notable WHO environmental-risk research projects focus on asthma in children and on the effects of arsenic poisoning during pregnancy on children.

Through the efforts of the Children's Environmental Health program, many countries have begun to identify and assess the environmental influences that affect the health and development of their youngest citizens. Many low- and middle-income countries have prepared a children's environmental health profile. These profiles provide a sound basis for countries and communities to set priorities for action, to plan appropriate environmental health programs, and to evaluate the progress that they have made.

WHO's Department of Child and Adolescent Health and Development promotes the health, growth, and development of young people from birth to age 19. It strives to speed up efforts by nations to improve the health and development of their young populations. The department has developed 25 strategies to achieve its goals. This enables each country to choose a strategy that is most appropriate for its specific needs. The department's major goals are to reduce the rate of infant and child deaths and the rate of HIV infection among people aged 15 to 24. The department has one of WHO's largest research programs. It supported two medical studies that examined potential treatments for pneumonia that could be administered in patients' homes in developing countries. The department also works with external partners. For example, it joined with UNICEF to develop a field manual for community-based health-care workers to use when treating severe malnutrition.

With the help of these WHO programs—and others— some countries have made remarkable progress. In 2007, global child deaths reached a record low, falling to 9.7 million. (Representing a drop to 68 deaths per 1,000 live births in 2007.) Excellent progress was made in many countries, included Bangladesh, Bolivia, Laos, Malawi, Niger, and Vietnam. These countries are on course to reach their child mortality reduction targets by 2015. Basic public health measures have had a major impact on these improvements. These measures have included measles immunizations, the use of insecticide-treated nets to prevent malaria, and programs to improve nutrition, sanitation, and water quality.

IMPROVE MATERNAL HEALTH

More than a half million women worldwide die each year during pregnancy and childbirth—about 1,500 deaths every day. In sub-Saharan Africa, for example, 6 percent of women are at risk of dying during pregnancy or childbirth over a lifetime. In comparison, only 1 in 2,800 women in wealthy countries face the same risk. Millennium Development Goal 5 seeks to improve maternal health to lower the number of deaths of mothers and their infants. One of the goal's targets is to reduce the maternal mortality rate between 1990 and 2015 by three-quarters. Most women who die in childbirth do so because there is not enough skilled primary and emergency care available where they live.

 A SUCCESS STORY

Each year, more than 400,000 women die during childbirth in sub-Saharan Africa. One country has started an innovative training program to help lower maternal death rates. In Mozambique, about 10 percent of women died during childbirth in 1992. By 2008, the nation's maternal death rate had dropped to less than 5 percent.

In 2004, the government launched a new program to train midwives to perform cesarean sections and other emergency childbirth surgeries. (A cesarean section is a surgical delivery of a baby that involves making cuts in the mother's abdomen and uterus.) Surgeons usually perform these types of operations, but Mozambique has only three doctors for every 100,000 people. By training midwives to perform these surgeries, the country has been able to provide more mothers with medical services during childbirth, particularly in rural

WHO's first major effort to improve maternal and newborn health started with its Safer Motherhood Initiative. Launched in 1987, this program partnered with other international agencies to address maternal mortality. Through the initiative, several countries made significant progress in reducing deaths among mothers and their newborns. Mother and child mortality, however, did not drop in many other countries. In response to the Millennium Development Goals, WHO reorganized the Safer Mother Initiative. Its new program, the Making Pregnancy Safer Initiative, increased WHO's efforts to improve mother and newborn health.

In 2005, WHO expanded the Making Pregnancy Safer Initiative, creating a new department to oversee the organization's work on maternal health. The Department of Making Pregnancy Safer assists countries to ensure that mothers

areas hundreds of miles from the nearest hospital. The midwives go through intensive training. One midwife, Emilia Cumbane, noted, "I think it's a good profession—to produce people."* The Mozambique midwife-surgery program shows how low-cost, community-based programs can improve public health in low-income countries. WHO's director-general, Dr. Margaret Chan, observed that the Mozambique program "is a story of courage. It is a story of innovation."**

* "Wide Angle: Birth of a Surgeon—Midwives in Mozambique." PBS. Available online at www.pbs.org/wnet/wideangle/episodes/birth-of-a-surgeon/introduction/747/.
** "Wide Angle: Birth of a Surgeon: Aaron Brown Interview: Dr. Margaret Chan." PBS. Available online at www.pbs.org/wnet/wideangle/episodes/birth-of-a-surgeon/aaron-brown-interview-dr-margaret-chan/1810/.

receive skilled care before, during, and after pregnancy and childbirth. The department also works to strengthen national health systems to provide mother and child care. WHO provides guidelines for safe pregnancy and childbirth and encourages countries to use them. These guidelines may save the lives of as many as 400,000 women each year. In some parts of the world, such as North Africa and Southeast Asia, more pregnant women now have greater access to health care. The department has staff working in more than 75 countries.

THE OTHER GOALS

Besides taking on a major role in meeting the Millennium Development Goals focused on health, WHO has accepted responsibility to assist global efforts to achieve the other goals. The WHO staff is working with member nations and other international agencies to eradicate extreme poverty and hunger, achieve universal primary education, promote gender equality and empower women, ensure environmental sustainability, and develop a global partnership for development. Some WHO efforts, such as its work to strengthen health-care systems worldwide, have an impact on more than one of the millennium goals.

Eradicate Extreme Poverty and Hunger

To fulfill Millennium Development Goal 1, the United Nations has established two targets. One target is to halve, by 2015, the proportion of people who suffer from hunger. WHO assists in achieving this target by focusing on two specific population groups. First, it works to reduce the percentage of underweight children younger than age five. Second, WHO works to reduce the percentage of people who regularly consume less than the average recommended daily nutrition requirement.

Nutrition is a key factor in good health and normal childhood development. Malnutrition makes people more vulnerable to infection and disease. Better nutrition contributes to better health. Healthy people are stronger and more productive. Programs that improve the nutrition of poor people can help them establish a better quality of life. WHO has collaborating centers for nutrition in 14 countries, including Brazil, Canada, France, Iran, Thailand, and Tanzania. These centers cooperate with other WHO personnel at the global, regional, and national levels. The centers promote all WHO policies related to nutrition. They collect information on good nutrition and distribute it to local people. They also provide nutrition training to health-care workers and work with other WHO departments on nutrition research.

Achieve Universal Primary Education

One of the targets in Millennium Development Goal 2 is to ensure that, by 2015, children everywhere will be able to complete a full course of primary schooling. Good health plays a crucial role in the ability of students to complete their primary schooling. Healthy children learn better. WHO's Global School Health Initiative was launched in 1995. It works to strengthen health promotion and education activities at all levels, from local to global. The initiative is designed to improve the health of students, school personnel, families, and other members of the community through school health programs.

In response to the Millennium Declaration, the Global School Health Initiative began to focus on increasing the number of health-promoting schools. WHO defines a health-promoting school as one that is "constantly strengthening its capacity as a healthy setting for living, learning, and working."[10] WHO has worked with such international agencies as UNESCO (United Nations Educational, Scientific, and Cultural Organization), UNAIDS (the Joint United Nations Program on HIV/AIDS), and the United States' Centers for Disease Control and Prevention to build regional networks to develop health-promoting schools. WHO also conducts research on ways to improve school health programs. It also works with national health and educational agencies to develop programs to improve student health. For example, WHO helped China create a program educating students about HIV/AIDS and other sexually transmitted diseases.

Promote Gender Equality and Empower Women

Millennium Development Goal 3 commits nations to promote gender equality and empower women. Women need special attention in health because they have unique health problems and risks. In addition, improving the health of women is an effective way to improve the health and prosperity of entire families. Healthy women can better care for their families and maintain employment.

In 2007, the World Health Assembly passed a resolution to make sure that gender issues were considered in all of the organization's work. WHO is helping to achieve this millennium goal by working to ensure gender equality in health-care services worldwide. WHO defines gender equality as "the absence of discrimination —on the basis of a person's sex—in providing opportunities, in allocating resources and benefits, or in access to services."[11] WHO's Gender, Women, and Health program focuses on increasing knowledge about biological, social, and cultural issues that have an impact on health. Because women face unequal access to health care in almost all countries, the Gender, Women, and Health program seeks to increase awareness about how gender affects health and to develop policies that increase gender equality in health.

Ensure Environmental Sustainability

To fulfill Millennium Development Goal 7, the UN has set as two of its targets to cut in half the proportion of people without sustainable access to safe drinking water and sanitation by 2015 and to achieve a significant improvement in the lives of at least 100 million slum dwellers by 2020. Environmental hazards, like unsafe water and air pollution, are responsible for about one-fourth of all diseases worldwide. In developing countries, the main diseases caused by environmental factors are malaria, diarrheal diseases, lower respiratory infections, and injuries. In developed countries, healthier environments could lower the number of cases of cancer, cardiovascular diseases, asthma, and other diseases.

WHO estimates that as many as 13 million deaths could be prevented each year by making the world's environments healthier. WHO's Public Health and Environment program works on a wide range of projects to improve environmental health. It promotes projects to provide safe water, improve hygiene, and adopt cleaner and safer home fuels. Other projects focus on increasing the safety of buildings, improving chemical safety, and reducing air pollution and the harmful effects of electromagnetic fields and ultraviolet radiation. The program also sponsors research on the effect of global environmental change on health.

Building a Global Partnership for Development

One target in Millennium Development Goal 8 is to provide access to affordable, essential drugs in developing countries. WHO's Health and Development program has helped nations establish their own lists of essential medicines. Most countries have developed these lists, but 19 developing nations have yet to create one or update their outdated list. An essential-medicines list contains those drugs that would satisfy the medical needs of most of the people in a country; these drugs should be available and affordable. WHO also provides assistance to nations in drafting medicine policies to govern the sale of essential drugs.

Several countries have made remarkable progress toward improving the affordability of essential drugs to combat HIV/AIDS, malaria, and tuberculosis. WHO continues to work with partners to provide access to essential drugs in developing countries. For example, in 2001, the organization

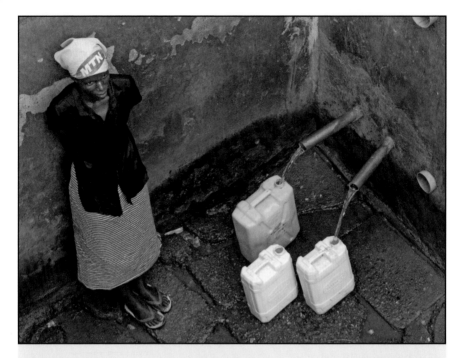

Experts estimate that the number of children dying unnecessarily from infectious diseases could be reduced by 2 million if good sanitation and water supplies were provided. WHO predicts that by 2015, 2.1 billion will still lack basic sanitation, and at the present rate sub-Saharan Africa will not reach the target until 2076. Above, a woman fills jugs with water at a water distribution point in the Naguru Go Down Slum in Kampala.

partnered with a Swiss pharmaceutical company to provide people in several countries with an antimalarial medicine at a significantly reduced price.

PROGRESS TOWARD THE GOALS

The Millennium Development Goals have had a major impact on the policies and work of WHO, other UN agencies, international organizations, and developing countries. Progress, however, has been slow. The health-related goals and targets that WHO embraced are unlikely to be achieved in many parts of the world.

To meet the goals, the health-care systems of developing countries need to be strengthened substantially. Without better health-care systems, countries cannot provide adequate programs for disease prevention and control. The resources needed to make effective improvements, however, are not available in most of these nations. The Millennium Declaration asked for wealthy countries to make a commitment to provide higher levels of aid. A significant percentage of this aid has yet to be donated. A worldwide economic crisis that struck in 2008 hit wealthy nations particularly hard. It has hindered their ability to meet aid commitments. Even if efforts to achieve the health-related millennium goals fall short of the objectives established in 2000, WHO's efforts will have made a meaningful difference in the lives of millions of people in the world's poorest countries.

Combating HIV/AIDS, Malaria, and Tuberculosis

MOST PEOPLE KNOW ABOUT WHO BECAUSE OF ITS WORLD-wide efforts to prevent, control, and eradicate infectious diseases. It has developed key programs to combat the threats to global public health posed by a wide range of infectious diseases. WHO also plays a central role in achieving the objectives of UN Millennium Development Goal 6. This goal seeks to halt, by 2015, the spread of HIV/AIDS, malaria, and tuberculosis and to begin to reverse their spread.

HIV/AIDS

The human immunodeficiency virus, or HIV, is a type of retrovirus. Retroviruses are particularly dangerous because they can make copies of themselves inside healthy cells that they have invaded. The HIV retrovirus attacks many different types of cells. Most importantly, it can harm T-helper lymphocytes and other cells that make up the human immune system. By invading these cells, HIV weakens the body's own defense against diseases.

HIV is transmitted through bodily fluids. The primary means of transmission is through sexual contact. Intravenous drug users who share needles also face a high risk of contracting the virus. HIV can be transmitted via transfusions of blood. (This is rare in developed countries, where blood is screened for HIV before being used.) HIV can also be passed from a mother to an infant during pregnancy, childbirth, and breastfeeding. The chance of this type of transmission is as high as 25 percent before and during childbirth and slightly higher through breastfeeding.

Scientists believe that HIV originated in sub-Saharan Africa. It spread to the Caribbean and then to the United States and Europe. They think that viruses in monkeys that weaken their immune systems mutated to HIV in humans who ate monkey meat. The first reports of a rare and deadly form of pneumonia appeared in 1981. Within a few years, AIDS had become widespread and was recognized as a specific disease.

In more than half of HIV cases, the infection is not detected in the early stages. The symptoms are often too mild to be noticed. These symptoms include fever, muscle aches, sore throat, a red rash, and a swelling of lymph glands. It can take 10 years or more for a person infected with HIV to notice major symptoms. As the infection slowly progresses, however, the person's immune system becomes weaker. That makes a person more vulnerable to infections, such as tuberculosis and influenza.

Once under control in most of the world, tuberculosis has made a dramatic comeback in the past two decades. A person with HIV is 20 times more likely to contract tuberculosis. Tuberculosis is the leading cause of death among those with HIV/AIDS. As AIDS spreads, so does tuberculosis. As much

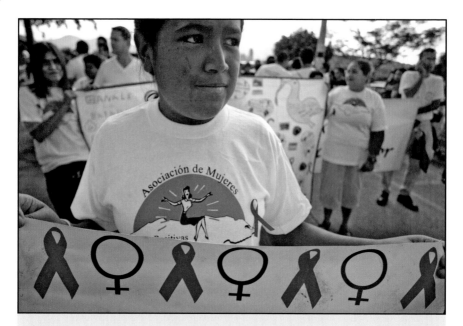

Although a 2008 study found that the death rates for HIV-infected patients decreased dramatically after the introduction of antiretroviral (ART) drugs, AIDS activists warn against complacency and ask that governments fill a multibillion dollar funding gap. Experts expect that in 2015 there will be 40,000 orphans in Honduras if preventive measures are not taken now. Above, members of Asociacíon de Mujeres march during World AIDS Day in Tegacigalpa, Honduras.

as one-third of the world's people may carry the tuberculosis bacteria. Each year, an estimated 2 million people a year die from the disease.

The most advanced stage of HIV infection is called acquired immunodeficiency syndrome, or AIDS. HIV infection becomes AIDS when the cells in a person's immune system have been destroyed. The AIDS epidemic has killed more than 25 million people. The number of people living with HIV in 2007 was 33 million. More than half were women. A new HIV infection occurs about every 15 seconds. Today, the rate of new HIV infections is rising more quickly among heterosexuals.

HIV/AIDS has its greatest impact in developing countries. Ninety-five percent of new infections occur in developing countries. Africa has the largest number of cases, but the infection rate is climbing in South Asia and Southeast Asia. The disease reveals the health-care disparity between rich and poor nations. In the poorest countries, people with HIV/AIDS often die without any medical care. Surveys in countries where HIV/AIDS is growing have found that as many as 90 percent of teens have never even heard of the disease. In wealthier countries, HIV/AIDS patients have access to antiretroviral drugs. These medications can slow down the development of AIDS and dramatically improve the lives of HIV/AIDS patients.

In the United States, HIV has spread from large cities to small towns and rural areas. AIDS was once the leading cause of death for Americans aged 25 to 44. It now ranks second after accidents. Antiretroviral drugs and other therapies have reduced the number of AIDS-related deaths in the United States and other developed countries.

Millions of deaths could be prevented in poor countries by using these drugs and therapies.

WHO's HIV/AIDS Efforts

WHO is a key player in the global effort to halt and reverse the spread of HIV/AIDS. Within the Joint United Nations Program on HIV/AIDS, known as UNAIDS, WHO is responsible for the global health response to the disease. WHO's primary goal is to enable member nations to make a comprehensive and sustainable health response to HIV/AIDS within their borders.

The task of halting and reversing the spread of HIV/AIDS is daunting. Nearly 3 million new cases of HIV/AIDS are diagnosed each year. More than 2 million people die of diseases related to HIV/AIDS each year. Only about 20 percent of people at high risk of HIV infection have access to the information and tools needed to prevent infection. Millions of HIV/AIDS patients are in urgent need of antiretroviral drugs.

WHO supports a public health approach to HIV prevention, treatment, care, and support. To accomplish this goal, WHO works with countries to develop straightforward treatment guidelines, decentralize health-care services, and give less-specialized health workers a larger role in treatment, care, and support.

WHO staff in all six regional offices and in 193 countries provide technical support and develop standards to prevent HIV/AIDS and to treat patients. The prevention programs seek to provide information, change behaviors to reduce HIV risks, and distribute condoms and sterile needles. WHO staff also train local health workers and provide advice on the most effective treatments. The most effective way to fight AIDS, WHO believes, is to increase the involvement of local communities and strengthen primary health-care services. WHO works to increase patients' access to treatments. WHO's AIDS Medicines and Diagnostic Services team helps member nations acquire and distribute affordable drugs and other medical supplies.

WHO's HIV/AIDS Department is its unit dedicated to preventing and controlling HIV/AIDS. It develops HIV/AIDS policies and guidelines, and supports nations in strengthening their capabilities to combat HIV/AIDS and acquiring HIV medications. It also monitors the global spread of HIV/AIDS and promotes greater attention to the epidemic.

Different teams within the HIV/AIDS Department work in specific areas of expertise. Among these teams are Antiretroviral Treatment and HIV Care, Systems Strengthening and HIV, and Strategic Information and Research. The HIV/AIDS Department is a member of the Cluster for HIV/AIDS, Tuberculosis, Malaria and Neglected Tropical Diseases.

The HIV/AIDS Department works closely with other WHO departments, programs, and teams. More than 30 other WHO departments carry out HIV/AIDS-related projects, including those working in the areas of blood safety, disease surveillance, sexual and reproductive health, and health education. These departments collaborate with other UN agencies, international development agencies, national health ministries, and local health-care providers in HIV/AIDS-related work. WHO's broad goal is to improve HIV prevention programs, enable people to know their HIV status, increase access to treatment and care, and strengthen national and local health systems.

WHO's Child and Adolescent Health and Development program works to prevent mother-to-child transmission of HIV, improve the care and treatment of infants with HIV

 MAKING A DIFFERENCE

Deepak and Rosy Khadgi, an HIV-positive couple in Nepal, started a nonprofit organization, Sahara Plus, to offer counseling and other services to HIV-positive people. They visit schools to talk to young people about sex, drugs, and AIDS. They also distribute antiretroviral drugs to HIV-positive patients who travel to their village from rural areas to pick up their medications.

Deepak was diagnosed with HIV in 1990. The couple has been married since 1995. They have two children who are HIV-negative. To fund Sahara Plus, Deepak makes and sells paintings that depict village life in his country. "My wife and I have been through a lot of pain, mostly because of the people who shunned us and shooed us away," he said. "We're not very educated. But we know enough about life that helping others is a kind of art. While I'm alive, I need to do as much as I can for as many people as I can."*

* *Portraits of Commitment: Why People Become Leaders in AIDS Work.* Bangkok, Thailand: Asia Pacific Leadership Forum on HIV/AIDS and Development, 2007, p. 59. Available online at *www.aplfaids.com/documents/SA_Portraits_book.pdf.*

infection, and prevent HIV in teens. The Stop TB Department integrates HIV/AIDS into its tuberculosis prevention and care programs. The Immunization, Vaccines, and Biologicals Department supports research to develop HIV vaccines. The Reproductive Health and Research Department works to include HIV/AIDS in programs to prevent and control sexually transmitted infections, and it supports research on improving the reliability of condoms. The Essential Health Technologies Department provides advice on blood transfusion safety and health-care worker protection.

In 2008, WHO produced a comprehensive collection of recommendations titled *Priority Interventions: HIV/AIDS Prevention, Treatment, and Care in the Health Sector*. Published as a book, CD-ROM, and Web site, the package described the most important and up-to-date policies and methods that politicians, public health officials, and health-care workers can use to tackle HIV/AIDS in their countries. WHO designed *Priority Interventions* to help low- and middle-income countries achieve broad access to HIV/AIDS prevention, treatment, and care services.

Millennium Development Goal 6 and HIV

The UN's Millennium Development Goal 6 committed the world's nations to combat HIV/AIDS and other diseases. WHO, in its primary role in coordinating global HIV/AIDS efforts, has two targets. The first is to halt and begin to reverse the spread of HIV/AIDS by 2015. The second is to achieve, by 2010, universal access to treatment for HIV/AIDS for all those who need it.

WHO monitors several health indicators to track the success of global HIV/AIDS efforts. For instance, WHO sponsors studies that assess HIV among young pregnant women (aged 15 to 24) and the rate of condom use.

WHO's efforts have resulted in progress in some areas. Its work to strengthen national prevention programs has lowered the number of new HIV cases. Its HIV prevention programs have successfully reduced risky sexual behaviors in many parts of the world. For example, the rate of global condom use has increased. The global growth of antiretroviral treatment services has also lowered the number of AIDS-related deaths worldwide.

Despite these victories, HIV/AIDS continues to take a terrible human toll, especially in sub-Saharan Africa. More than 7,000 people worldwide become infected with HIV each day. More than 5,000 people a day die from AIDS. The rate of women contracting HIV infection is increasing worldwide. The greater effectiveness and wider availability of antiretroviral drugs and other HIV/AIDS treatments has resulted in many patients living longer lives. The number of people living with HIV increased from 29.5 million in 2001 to 33 million in 2007. Many national health systems, however, cannot handle the treatment and care needs of larger numbers of HIV/AIDS survivors. Predicting the future of AIDS is difficult. It will continue to be one of the most critical challenges facing global public health.

MALARIA

Malaria is a serious infectious disease that occurs most frequently in tropical climates. It is caused by four specific species of parasites. *Plasmodium falciparum* (the deadliest form) and *Plasmodium vivax* are the two most common types. About 40 percent of the world's population faces the threat of malaria. Most people at risk live in the world's poorest countries.

More than 500 million people become ill with malaria each year. Most cases and deaths occur in sub-Saharan Africa. The disease also occurs in Asia, the Middle East, Latin America, and some parts of Europe. Malaria presents different threats to different countries. Some regions of the world have a steady number of malaria cases throughout the year. Other areas experience malaria cases only during certain parts of the year, usually during a rainy season.

Widespread malaria epidemics can erupt in regions where people have had little or no exposure to malaria. These epidemics are usually caused by unusual weather conditions that expand the range of mosquito populations. Disasters or other events can also lead to malaria epidemics when large numbers of people move into regions with malaria. Travelers from countries that do not experience malaria are always particularly at risk.

Mosquitoes spread malaria among humans. When a female mosquito bites a person with malaria, it ingests blood containing the malaria parasites. When the mosquito bites another person, it passes the malaria parasites into that person's bloodstream. Once in the bloodstream, the parasites travel to the person's liver. There, they multiply quickly and re-enter the bloodstream in huge numbers. By the time symptoms appear, thousands of parasites have clogged blood vessels and caused blood cells to burst. Malaria symptoms include chills alternating with fever, fatigue, headache, nausea, and an enlarged spleen.

Malaria can be treated and prevented with a wide variety of medications, including chloroquine and mefloquin. Early diagnosis and immediate treatment help control the disease and prevent life-threatening complications from developing. If left untreated, malaria can disrupt the blood supply to the body's organs. In many parts of the world, the malaria parasites have developed resistance to antimalarial drugs. These new drug-resistant strains pose a serious threat to global public health.

Malaria results in enormous social and economic costs in countries where it is endemic (common in a particular location). It lowers job and school attendance, contributes to poverty, and discourages foreign investment and tourism. WHO estimates that malaria causes an average drop of more than 1 percent of economic growth in countries with large-scale malaria problems. Over the years, this loss has resulted in significant differences in economic output between nations with malaria and those without. Low-income countries hit hard by malaria struggle to control or eliminate the disease. A large percentage of their public health budgets is directed toward malaria treatment and prevention.

WHO's Malaria Efforts

WHO's Global Malaria Program coordinates its efforts to combat malaria worldwide. The program provides member nations with advice on policy and strategies to prevent, control, and treat malaria. It recommends that countries adopt four malaria strategies:

1. Prevention through techniques that protect against mosquito bites.
2. Immediate treatment of malaria with effective drugs.
3. Special focus on protecting young children and pregnant women.
4. Strengthening national capacities to detect and react to malaria epidemics.

The specific malaria policies appropriate for a nation will depend on many factors. The type of malaria (parasite species), patterns of disease transmission, the prevalence of drug-resistant strains, and various political and economic issues must be considered in order to develop an effective and affordable national malaria program.

The Global Malaria Program also participates in the Roll Back Malaria Partnership. Created in 1998, the partnership's goal is to reduce malaria worldwide so that it no longer is a major cause of death or a major obstacle to economic development. It works to promote increased investment in national health systems in order to provide effective malaria prevention and treatment to populations most at risk. The partnership supports

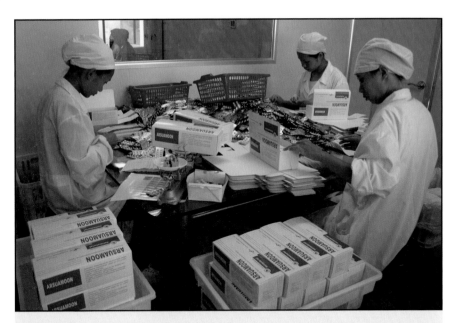

Employees in Guilin, China, wrap the malaria drug artesumate for exporting. WHO listed the artesumate injection by the Guilin Pharmaceutical Company as the first choice in emergency treatment for malaria. The company is the only producer of the drug in China that has met WHO requirements. It has kept the price of the drug in Africa, a region that suffers worst from malaria, at only 60 percent of the cost for pharmaceuticals produced by Western companies.

research into new and more effective tools (including a promising vaccine that is being developed) against malaria. Besides WHO, partners include the United Nations Development Program, UNICEF, the World Bank, nations, foundations, research institutions, and privately owned companies.

Millennium Development Goal 6 and Malaria

The UN's Millennium Development Goal 6 committed the world's nations to combat malaria and other diseases. WHO plays a primary role in coordinating global malaria efforts.

WHO's target is to halt and begin to reverse the spread of malaria by 2015. To measure its progress toward this target, WHO closely monitors two global health indicators: (1) malaria's prevalence and death rate and (2) the percentage of people in at-risk areas who are using effective prevention and treatment measures.

A 2008 UN report concluded that more progress had been made in treating malaria than in preventing it. New malaria treatment strategies are effective but have not expanded adequately into high-risk regions. The report also noted an encouraging increase in the use of insecticide-treated mosquito nets in high-risk regions, lowering the infection rate. The global distribution of mosquito nets, however, fell short of UN goals. WHO has achieved success in some malaria regions. In South Africa's KwaZulu-Natal province, for example, malaria cases plunged by 90 percent from 2000 to 2004. Several factors contributed to this remarkable achievement, including health education, a government program to spray indoors with pesticides, and the commitment and hard work of the national government, community groups, and international agencies.

TUBERCULOSIS

Tuberculosis, or TB, is a serious infectious respiratory disease that primarily affects the lungs. A bacteria, *Mycobacterium tuberculosis*, causes the disease. An infection that solely affects the lungs is known as pulmonary tuberculosis. An infection that starts in the lungs sometimes spreads to other parts of the body, including bones, joints, blood vessels, kidneys, ovaries, and skin.

Tuberculosis is spread when an infected person coughs, sneezes, or exhales. Tiny droplets containing the tuberculosis bacteria are released into the air. People nearby can inhale the droplets into their nasal passages and lungs. An infected person may show various symptoms, including a persistent cough, loss of appetite, chest pains, and difficulty breathing. Tuberculosis is not highly contagious. It usually requires close or prolonged contact to be transmitted. The immune systems of healthy people usually prevent the bacterial infection from spreading.

About 9 million new cases of tuberculosis are reported each year. Worldwide, a new infection occurs every second. The disease kills about 2 million people annually. Over the next 20 years, a billion people are likely to become infected with tuberculosis; 35 million will die from it. About one-third of the world's population is already infected with the tuberculosis bacteria. Only 5 to 10 percent of people with tuberculosis ever become sick or infectious. People with HIV/AIDS, however, are particularly vulnerable to tuberculosis infections. They have a 20-times greater chance of acquiring the disease. Regional increases in tuberculosis cases have mirrored regional increases in HIV/AIDS.

WHO's Tuberculosis Efforts

WHO has several programs and partnerships that help member nations build health systems to prevent, treat, and cure tuberculosis. The organization began its Stop TB Strategy in 2006. The key element of the strategy is DOTS (which stands for directly observed treatment, short-course), WHO's long-running tuberculosis-control program. Since 1995, DOTS-related programs have treated more than 22 million patients worldwide. Through the Stop TB Strategy, WHO seeks to expand and enhance the DOTS program, find new approaches to preventing and combating tuberculosis in HIV/AIDS patients, and support new research on tuberculosis.

The Stop TB Strategy has made good progress toward its DOTS targets. It is very close to achieving the target percentage of new cases to be treated under DOTS. The program has also nearly met its treatment success rate target. Although cure rates in Africa and Eastern Europe were lower, the average DOTS cure rate is about 85 percent. WHO's 2007 *Global TB Control Report* showed that 26 countries had met their DOTS targets, including China and Vietnam, two nations with high numbers of tuberculosis cases. WHO believes that the number of worldwide tuberculosis cases peaked in 2005. It remains confident that, if the Stop TB Strategy continues to be implemented, infections and deaths can be cut in half by 2015 in all regions of the world except Africa and Eastern Europe.

WHO is the lead agency of the Stop TB Partnership. Established in 2000, the partnership seeks to eliminate tuberculosis as a public health threat. Its key mission is to make sure that every tuberculosis patient has access to effective medical care and treatment. It also works to stop the transmission of tuberculosis by developing new policies and public health approaches to the disease. Other partners include the United Nations Development Program, UNAIDS, many nations, and international agencies.

In 2008, the Stop TB Partnership published *Luìs Figo and the World Tuberculosis Cup*, a comic book that informs teens about tuberculosis and how to prevent it. In the comic book, real-life Portuguese soccer star Luìs Figo captains the teenaged Stop Tuberculosis Team, which plays against a team of tuberculosis germs. In a statement released when the comic book was published, Figo urged young people to take its message seriously: "Tuberculosis is a killer, and I want all of you to stay safe from it. I am passing the ball to you—you can help reach the goal of stopping tuberculosis."[12]

WHO has joined with other international agencies and organizations in the TB/HIV Working Group. The group develops policies and methods to control HIV-related tuberculosis. It supports cooperation between organizations and people fighting against tuberculosis and those fighting against HIV/AIDS. This collaboration will help HIV patients avoid tuberculosis infection and improve services to HIV patients who have contracted tuberculosis.

The main challenge facing WHO in achieving its tuberculosis target is the rise of drug-resistant strains of the disease.

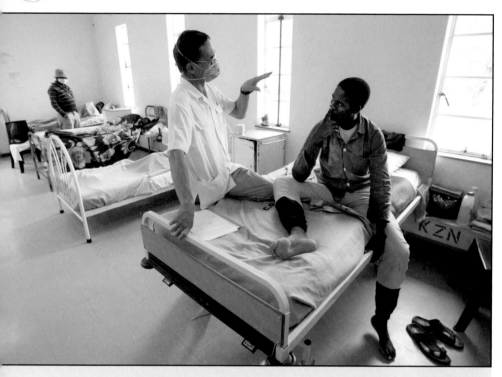

Successful diagnosis of extensively drug-resistant tuberculosis (XDR-TB) relies on the patients' access to quality health-care services. Since this new strain of the disease emerged from the mismanagement of treatment and improper diagnosis, WHO fears that XDR-TB could become a major killer in parts of Africa hit hardest by AIDS where governments have been slow to roll out TB control programs.

These new strains have become increasingly difficult to treat because all of the major anti-tuberculosis drugs have little effect on them. The drug-resistant strains appear to be spreading. Drug-resistant tuberculosis can be treated with chemotherapy, a much more invasive and expensive treatment.

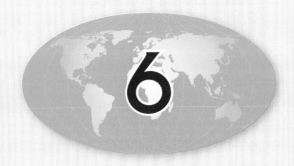

Preventing and Controlling Chronic Diseases

CHRONIC DISEASES ARE ILLNESSES THAT HAVE LONG DURATIONS and are usually never completely cured. Heart attacks, strokes, cancer, diabetes, and asthma are the most common types. Chronic diseases are the leading cause of death in the world, accounting for 60 percent of all deaths. In developed countries, they make up as much as 70 percent of all deaths. WHO has documented a troubling trend in the global surge of chronic diseases. They are causing an increasing percentage of deaths in developing countries. About 80 percent of all deaths from chronic diseases now occur in developing countries. A 2008 WHO publication noted, "As populations age in middle- and low-income countries over the next 25 years, the proportion of deaths due to [chronic] diseases will rise significantly."[13]

Each year, about 17 million people die from chronic diseases. Three major factors—unhealthy diet, a lack of physical activity, and tobacco use—underlie many chronic diseases. If these factors were controlled or eliminated, as much as 80 percent of heart disease, stroke, and diabetes cases could be prevented. Likewise, 30 percent of cancer cases could be prevented. To protect the health of people worldwide, several WHO departments and programs focus on preventing and controlling chronic diseases.

CARDIOVASCULAR DISEASES

Cardiovascular diseases are a group of several diseases that afflict the heart and other parts of the circulatory system. Coronary heart disease (which can result in a heart attack) and cerebrovascular disease (which can result in a stroke) are the two most common types of cardiovascular disease. Blockages that prevent blood from flowing to the heart or the brain are the main causes of heart attacks and strokes, respectively. Blood clots or build-ups of fatty deposits inside blood vessels typically cause these blockages. Other types of cardiovascular diseases include peripheral arterial disease, rheumatic heart disease, and congenital heart disease.

The primary risk factors that lead to cardiovascular diseases are unhealthy diets, lack of physical activity, and use of tobacco products. Other risk factors include poverty, stress, and aging. These factors often lead to high blood pressure, high blood-sugar levels, and obesity. Cardiovascular diseases often have no symptoms until a heart attack or a stroke occurs.

Cardiovascular diseases are the number one cause of death worldwide, making up about 25 percent of all deaths. WHO estimates that nearly 8 million people a year die from heart attacks, and almost 6 million die from strokes annually. WHO projects that, by 2015, nearly 20 million people will die each year from cardiovascular diseases. Cardiovascular diseases also have a significant social and economic impact. They often strike middle-aged people, affecting their ability to work and threatening the finances of their families.

Through its Department of Chronic Disease and Health Promotion, WHO seeks to prevent early deaths and disability due to cardiovascular diseases. To achieve this goal, WHO staff works to help people worldwide avoid the factors that can lead to cardiovascular diseases. By changing people's health behaviors, about four out of five premature deaths from heart disease and stroke could be prevented. A person can greatly reduce the risk of suffering from a cardiovascular disease (as well as other chronic diseases) by:

- eating a healthy diet that includes plenty of fruits and vegetables and excludes foods high in salt, sugar, or fat.
- maintaining a healthy body weight.
- engaging in regular physical activity.
- avoiding tobacco smoke.

WHO offers national health agencies advice on how to adopt effective programs and policies to provide healthy meals for students, encourage physical activity, and control tobacco use. It also supports national efforts to improve access to affordable medications and medical devices that treat cardiovascular diseases. WHO supports efforts to raise awareness of the effects of cardiovascular diseases, particularly among poorer segments of national populations.

CANCER

Cancer is a group of nearly 100 diseases. All types of cancer share two key characteristics: uncontrolled growth of abnormal cells in the body and the ability of these cells to spread to other parts of the body. Cancer originates with a change in a single cell. External agents that can cause cancer—such as viruses, hormones, chemicals, or radiation—work together with hereditary

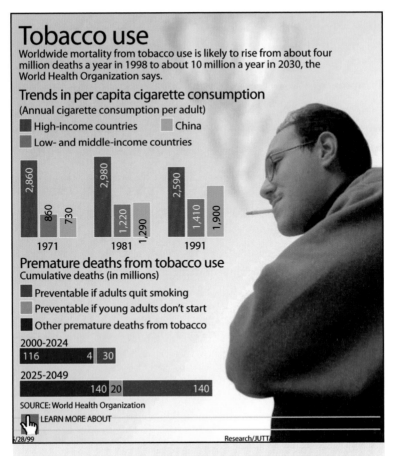

Tobacco use

Worldwide mortality from tobacco use is likely to rise from about four million deaths a year in 1998 to about 10 million a year in 2030, the World Health Organization says.

Trends in per capita cigarette consumption
(Annual cigarette consumption per adult)

■ High-income countries ■ China
■ Low- and middle-income countries

1971: 2,860, 860, 730
1981: 2,980, 1,220, 1,290
1991: 2,590, 1,410, 1,900

Premature deaths from tobacco use
Cumulative deaths (in millions)

■ Preventable if adults quit smoking
■ Preventable if young adults don't start
■ Other premature deaths from tobacco

2000-2024
116 | 4 | 30

2025-2049
140 | 20 | 140

SOURCE: World Health Organization

LEARN MORE ABOUT

5/28/99 Research/JUTTA

The theme for WHO's 20th World No Tobacco Day, held on May 31, 2009, was "Tobacco Health Warnings." Tobacco kills half of all who use it, yet it is common throughout the world due to its low cost, aggressive marketing, and inconsistent public policies against it. WHO approves of warnings incorporating both pictures and words because they have been shown to be most effective in getting users to quit.

factors to cause this cellular change. If the spread of abnormal cells is not controlled, it can result in death.

Tobacco use is the primary risk factor that leads to cancers. Other risk factors include aging, alcohol use, unhealthy diet, obesity, air pollution, and infections like HIV and hepatitis B.

These factors can trigger vital changes in the body, transforming a normal cell into a precancerous lesion and then into a malignant tumor.

Cancer has become one of the leading causes of death worldwide. It accounts for about 8 million deaths a year, or 13 percent of all deaths. WHO has documented that more than 80 percent of all cancer deaths occur in low- and middle-income countries. WHO projects that, by 2030, annual cancer deaths will rise to 10 million. Lung, stomach, liver, colon, and breast cancer are the types of cancer that cause the most deaths.

A 2005 cancer study concluded that about 30 percent of cancer deaths could be prevented if nations adopted bet-

CANCER TAKES ITS TOLL ON A FAMILY

In 2004, doctors told 45-year-old Miriame Nnamusoke that she had cervical cancer. The illness forced her to stop working as a farmer in her small village in Uganda. She went to a private hospital to receive treatment. Her life savings soon ran out, however, and she had to leave the hospital. Her daughter dropped out of school to care for her. Losing their home, they moved in with Miriame's brother in Kampala, the country's capital. He struggled to support his two sons, along with his sister and his niece.

Miriame received radiotherapy treatments in a Kampala hospital, but she was not cured. The disease had been diagnosed too late. Miriame's situation is common in many low-income countries, where basic screening for chronic diseases is not widely available. A nongovernmental organization, Hospice Africa-Uganda, sent a health-care worker to visit Miriame every two weeks. The worker provided counseling and pain-relief medication to ease Miriame's suffering until she died.

ter cancer-prevention methods and expanded early-detection programs. National prevention methods include providing guidance and incentives for people to avoid or reduce key risk factors, developing vaccination programs for the hepatitis B virus and other infectious diseases linked to cancer, and controlling environmental hazards at workplaces and in neighborhoods. Two important elements needed for effective early detection of cancer are:

1. education to help people recognize early signs of cancer and know when to seek medical care.
2. screening programs, such as mammograms to detect breast cancer, to identify early signs of cancer.

Early detection is important because the earlier a cancer is diagnosed, the more effective treatments are. The goal of early-detection programs is to find the cancer before it spreads to other parts of the body.

Many effective treatments exist to help cancer patients. Some types of cancer have high cure rates when detected early and treated through surgery, chemotherapy (a treatment that uses special chemicals), and other methods. These treatments typically require laboratory tests and such technologies as ultrasound and endoscopy. In places where medical resources are scarce, affordable treatments can prolong the lives of patients and improve their quality of life. Dr. Catherine Le Galès-Camus, WHO's assistant director-general for noncommunicable diseases and mental health, noted, "It is possible, even in very economically constrained environments, to be effective in preventing cancer and improving access to quality services for patients who need such services."[14]

To improve methods to prevent, cure, and treat cancer, WHO launched its Global Action Plan Against Cancer in 2007. The primary goal of the initiative is to help member nations develop their own national cancer programs. WHO seeks to include partners from both the public and private sectors and make sure that programs are integrated into other national public health programs. The agency stresses that these national cancer programs should not exclude poor people and should be cost-effective so that countries can afford to maintain the programs in the future. WHO provides support to nations to improve their primary health-care systems and their specialized treatment programs for cancer patients. It also supplies essential medicines and technologies for cancer treatment and patient care. WHO provides assistance to ensure that nations can adopt new cancer strategies and treatments as quickly as possible.

On the international level, WHO works with other UN agencies and other partners on broad projects to prevent and control cancer. It supports new cancer research and distributes the latest scientific evidence and information to member nations. WHO develops standards and practices to guide the planning and implementation of international programs for cancer prevention, early detection, and treatment.

In 2003, the World Health Assembly negotiated WHO's Framework Convention on Tobacco Control. The treaty sought to create effective programs to combat tobacco use. There are more than one billion smokers in the world. Tobacco is a risk factor for six of the eight leading causes of death. It kills about half of the people who use it, and tobacco smoke poses serious health risks to nonsmokers. Secondhand smoke causes cancer, heart disease, and many other serious illnesses. Nearly half of all children in the world breathe air polluted by tobacco smoke. The smoke makes their asthma conditions worse and causes dangerous diseases.

Tobacco use is the foremost preventable cause of death worldwide. It kills more than 5 million people a year, accounting for 10 percent of adult deaths annually. Tobacco use is growing worldwide. If the current trend continues, WHO projects that tobacco will kill more than 8 million people annually by 2030 and as many as a billion people during the twenty-first century.

Most tobacco use begins during adolescence. Today, more than 150 million teens use tobacco. WHO urges governments to protect the world's 1.8 billion young people by imposing a ban on all tobacco advertising and promotional and sponsorship efforts by tobacco companies. In 2008, Dr. Margaret Chan, WHO's director-general, declared, "Reversing this entirely preventable epidemic must now rank as a top priority for public health and for political leaders in every country of the world."[15]

OBESITY AND OVERWEIGHT

Obesity is an abnormal accumulation of body fat. Overweight is an excessive accumulation of fat. A measurement called body mass index (BMI) helps determine whether a person is obese or overweight. To calculate BMI, multiply a person's weight in pounds by 703 and then divide that number by the square of the person's height in inches. (In the metric system, BMI is calculated by dividing the person's weight in kilograms by the square of the person's height in meters.) BMI provides only a rough guide. It may not provide an accurate result because degrees of fatness vary among individuals. Some BMI charts, for example, have separate scales for men and women and separate ideal weight ranges for people of the same height who have different body frames (small, medium, and large).

WHO considers a person obese if he or she has a BMI equal to or more than 30. It considers a person overweight if she or he has a BMI of 25.0 to 29.9. Research has shown that the risk of chronic diseases begins to increase once a person's BMI reaches 21. About 1.6 billion adults (15 years old or older) worldwide are overweight. About 400 million adults are obese. WHO projects that, by 2015, as many as 2.3 billion adults will be overweight, and 700 million will be obese. In the past, obese and overweight people were mostly found in wealthy countries. Over the past decade, they have risen significantly in low- and middle-income countries. Adults are not the only people affected. More than 22 million children worldwide under five years old are overweight.

The primary cause of obesity and overweight is a person consuming more calories than he or she burns. The body stores excess calories as fat tissue. Researchers believe that genetic factors, psychological factors, and social factors contribute to weight gain. Some diseases, including hypothryoidism, and the use of steroids and certain other drugs can also cause weight gain.

Several factors have played a major role in the dramatic worldwide increase in people who are obese or overweight. Around the world, people's diets have changed. Many people now eat more foods that are high in sugars and fat. Many people have also become less physically active. Increased urbanization, the wider use of motorized transportation, and changes in the types of jobs (more people working in offices, for example) have contributed to a shift in many people's calorie balance.

Being obese or overweight can lead to serious health problems. Higher BMI is a risk factor for such chronic diseases as heart attack and stroke, diabetes, arthritis, and some cancers. It can also lead to high blood pressure, shortness of breath, pregnancy complications, sleeping disorders, and emotional and social problems. Studies have shown that obese children are more likely to die young or experience a disability when they become adults.

Obesity and overweight, and the chronic diseases related to them, are mostly preventable. People can reduce their BMIs by:

- limiting their intake of fats and sugars.
- eating more fruits, vegetables, whole grains, and nuts.
- increasing physical activity (a minimum of 30 minutes of moderately intense activity on most days is needed).

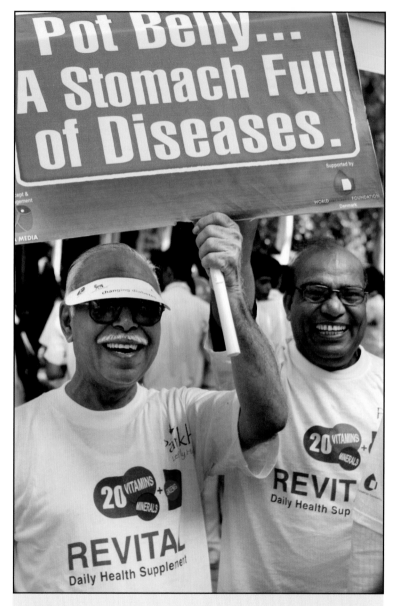

Obesity and overweight now affect 50 to 65 percent of the population, not only in North America, Europe, and Australia, but also in lower- to moderate-income countries. WHO estimates that India has about 37 million diabetes patients, and by the year 2025 it could reach 57.5 million. Above, men hold a banner during a walk advocating the prevention of obesity, diabetes, and heart diseases in New Delhi, India.

Through its Global Strategy on Diet, Physical Activity, and Health, WHO works to achieve worldwide adoption of healthy diets and regular physical activity. The Department of Chronic Diseases and Health Promotion leads WHO's efforts on diet and physical activity. It works with international partners, governments, and private enterprises to create healthier environments and make healthier diet options affordable and easily accessible. The department especially focuses on poor populations and children. Both of these groups often have limited options for what they can eat and where they can live.

WHO's Department of Nutrition for Health and Development also promotes healthy diets. It helps nations develop effective national nutrition policies and programs. The department also works with food industry companies to lower portion sizes and to reduce the fat, sugar, and salt content of processed foods.

DIABETES

Diabetes is a chronic disease that occurs when the pancreas no longer produces enough insulin or when cells stop responding to the insulin that the body produces. When the body digests foods that contain carbohydrates (sugars and starches), it produces a sugar known as glucose. Blood carries glucose throughout the body, supplying cells with the energy that they need to work properly. Insulin is a chemical that is produced by the pancreas, an organ located near the stomach. Insulin causes a chemical reaction that allows glucose carried in the bloodstream to flow into cells. When the pancreas does not produce enough insulin or when cells no longer respond to insulin, glucose remains in the bloodstream.

The body reacts to higher glucose levels in the blood by drawing water out of cells. The water helps the body expel the excess glucose through urine. Body cells become dried out and become starved for energy, triggering thirst and hunger cravings. To provide energy for cells, the body tries to convert fats and proteins to glucose. This leads to a life-threatening condition when acidic compounds called ketones build up in the blood.

There are two types of diabetes. Type 1 diabetes occurs when the pancreas does not produce enough insulin. It usually develops by the teen years. Without the daily administration of insulin, Type 1 is fatal. Type 2 diabetes occurs when the body does not use insulin effectively. About 90 percent of diabetics worldwide have Type 2, which primarily arises as a result of excess body weight and physical inactivity. It usually affects adults, but obese children are now being diagnosed with the disease.

WHO estimates that more than 180 million people worldwide suffer from diabetes. It projects that, by 2030, the number of diabetics may double. More than one million people die from diabetes each year. Nearly 80 percent of these deaths occur in low- and middle-income countries. Almost half of the people who die from diabetes are younger than 70 years old.

Diabetes causes many serious health problems and doubles a person's risk of dying. Diabetes can damage the heart and kidneys. About 70 percent of diabetics die from heart disease, stroke, or kidney failure. Diabetes can damage small blood vessels in the retina, leading to blindness. Research has shown that, after 15 years of diabetes, about 1 in 50 diabetics becomes blind. About 1 in 10 develops a serious impairment of their sight. Diabetes can also damage nerves, causing pain, numbness, or weakness in the feet and hands. Reduced blood flow can lead to amputations, particularly of the feet and legs.

Symptoms of diabetes include frequent urination, sluggishness, excessive thirst, and hunger. To help prevent Type 2 diabetes and its many threats to good health, people should:

- maintain a healthy body weight.
- engage in physical activity.
- have regular blood tests, which aid in diagnosing the disease at an early stage.
- stop using tobacco products.

Through its Diabetes Program, WHO supports countries in adopting effective measures to detect, prevent, and control diabetes. It provides scientific guidelines for diabetes prevention and develops standards for diabetes care. The Diabetes Program also draws attention to the health threats posed by diabetes, particularly through its partnership with the International Diabetes Federation. The two organizations sponsor World Diabetes Day, held each November 14 to raise awareness of diabetes. The Diabetes Program supports research and statistical studies on the disease and its risk factors. For example, one research project assessed how increased rates of obesity worldwide would affect the number of people with diabetes.

ASTHMA AND OTHER RESPIRATORY DISORDERS

Asthma is a long-lasting inflammatory disease of the air passages to and from the lungs. An inflammation of the lining of the bronchial tubes causes them to swell, reducing the flow of air into and out of the lungs. The narrowing of the airways results in wheezing, shortness of breath, and gasping for air. The inflammation sometimes stops spontaneously and can also be treated with a wide range of medications. Over time, the repeated inflammations make the airways particularly sensitive to cold air, dust, pollutants, and even stress. Similar respiratory disorders include chronic obstructive pulmonary disease, respiratory allergies, occupational lung diseases, and pulmonary hypertension.

About 300 million people worldwide suffer from asthma. More than 200 million people have chronic obstructive pulmonary disease and other chronic respiratory ailments. Asthma is the most common chronic disease among children. Compared with other chronic diseases, it has a low fatality rate. Most asthma-related deaths occur in low-income and lower-middle-income countries. Asthma can impair a person's daily activities for his or her entire life, however, and can cause such health problems as sleeplessness and constant fatigue.

The causes of asthma are not completely understood. Researchers believe that hereditary factors combine with environmental factors either to cause allergic reactions or to irritate the airways. Irritants include such inhaled substances as air pollution, pollen, dust mites, pet dander, mold, tobacco smoke, and chemicals. Intense emotions, such as anger and fear, and certain types of medicines (including aspirin) can trigger asthma attacks.

The severity and frequency of asthma symptoms vary among patients. Asthma attacks can occur several times a day or much less often. The factors that trigger asthma attacks also vary among patients. A cure has yet to be discovered, but asthma can be controlled. Medications can relieve short-term symptoms, such as wheezing. To control the underlying inflammation of the lining of the bronchial tubes, patients can take additional medication. They can also control their asthma by avoiding specific triggers.

Through its Chronic Respiratory Diseases Program, WHO coordinates international efforts to prevent and control asthma and other chronic respiratory disorders. It supports the efforts of member nations to reduce disability and premature death related to respiratory diseases. The program gathers information and statistics on respiratory diseases. It provides advice on establishing national prevention programs to reduce the level of exposure to common risk factors, particularly air pollution and tobacco smoke. The program also gives guidance on setting up strategies that provide affordable treatments and medications to patients with chronic respiratory diseases. Along with its international partners in the Global Alliance Against Chronic Respiratory Diseases, WHO helps low- and middle-income countries provide chronic respiratory-disease health services.

OTHER CHRONIC DISEASES AND INJURIES

WHO works to prevent and control other chronic diseases. Many types of chronic diseases, ranging from musculoskeletal

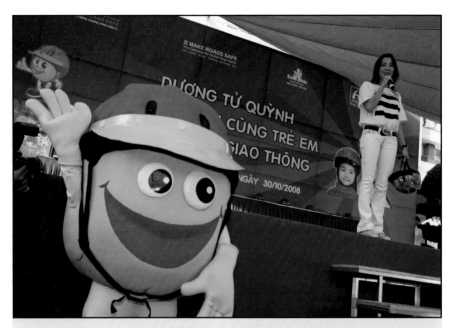

As of 2002, accidental injuries were blamed for the deaths of 1,000 children per week in Vietnam. The Helmets for Kids program has distributed helmets to 150,000 children in 100 schools. Here, film star and Road Safety Goodwill Ambassador Michelle Yeoh opens the ceremony for the start of the Decade of Action for Road Safety march in Ho Chi Minh City, Vietnam, in October 2008.

and oral disorders to digestive and skin diseases, account for about 9 percent of all deaths worldwide each year. WHO programs, such as the Global Oral Health Program, work to prevent and control specific chronic diseases. WHO teams are also dedicated to the prevention of blindness and visual impairment and deafness and hearing impairment.

Accidents and injuries kill more than 5 million people each year, accounting for 9 percent of all deaths. Traffic accidents, poisoning, drownings, falls, burns, and various forms of violence (acts of war and assaults) are major threats in all nations. Survivors often suffer temporary or permanent disabilities. WHO's Department of Violence and Injury Prevention and

Disability collects and analyzes data on accidents and injuries. It advises member nations on methods to build and improve health care and support services for victims of accidents and injuries. The rise in car ownership in rapidly developing countries, such as China and India, has caused the annual number of traffic fatalities to soar. In response, the department works with nations to design programs to prevent traffic deaths and injuries, including WHO's Helmet Initiative. The Helmet Initiative promotes the use of helmets as a way to prevent head injuries in bicycle and motorcycle accidents. The department also works to improve global emergency care and rehabilitation services.

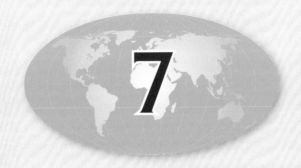

Ensuring Global Health

WHO'S MANY DEPARTMENTS AND PROGRAMS ARE DEDICATED to ensuring global public health. As part of that effort, the organization administers international health regulations that protect the world's people from infectious diseases. WHO's member nations have agreed to comply with a set of international health rules that help prevent the spread of diseases around the world. WHO has emergency-response units that provide assistance with epidemics and humanitarian health crises. It can offer immediate support and expertise when major public health emergencies arise. These units include WHO's Strategic Health Operations Center, the Global Outbreak Alert and Response Network, the Health Action in Crises program, and the Disease Control in Humanitarian Emergencies program.

INTERNATIONAL HEALTH REGULATIONS

WHO's International Health Regulations are a set of laws that help nations work together to prevent the spread of diseases and other health risks between countries. The World Health Assembly adopted the original regulations, known as International Sanitary Regulations, in 1951. These original regulations updated various international sanitary rules that had been adopted since the mid-1800s. They also brought together all of the existing rules of public health.

The 1951 regulations focused on monitoring and controlling six serious infectious diseases—cholera, plague, relapsing fever (a bacterial infection), smallpox, typhus, and yellow fever. The regulations required governments to notify WHO if an outbreak of any of these six diseases occurred within their borders. The 1951 rules also provided conditions under which vaccinations could be required as a condition for a person to enter a country. For example, many countries required (and still require today) visitors arriving from a country where yellow fever was present to show proof that they had received a yellow fever vaccination. Because modern modes of transportation allowed diseases to spread more easily, the 1951 regulations provided sanitary rules for all forms of transportation—ships, airplanes, trains, and motor vehicles. For example, one rule provided guidance on effective methods to rid ships of rats. (Rat fleas can transmit diseases like typhus and plague to humans.)

In 1969, the World Health Assembly revised these regulations and renamed them the International Health Regulations. The 1969 rules focused on preventing the spread of only four diseases: cholera, plague, smallpox, and yellow fever. Countries were no longer required to notify WHO of outbreaks of relapsing fever or typhus. Minor modifications to the regulations were made in 1973 and 1981.

2005 International Health Regulations

Representatives to the World Health Assembly recognized that the expansion of globalization increased the risks to human health. In 2005, the assembly approved a major overhaul of the International Health Regulations. Rapid growth in international travel and trade increased the likelihood that diseases could spread quickly around the world. Global trade increased the potential for food-borne diseases spreading beyond national borders. It also boosted the potential for contaminated drugs and other goods to be shipped worldwide.

The 2005 regulations went into effect in 2007. They established new sets of rules in three key areas. The first set required countries to improve their monitoring and reporting of public health events, such as disease outbreaks. The second set provided countries with guidelines to strengthen their ability to respond to public health events. The third set focused on helping countries expand their support of WHO's existing emergency-response programs.

The new rules required international notification for four diseases: polio, SARS, smallpox, and cases of influenza caused by any new subtype. The regulations urged countries to improve their ability to prevent and control disease outbreaks and also gave WHO a more direct role in investigating and stopping outbreaks. The rules empowered WHO to work closely with nations to make sure that they have the skills and personnel to meet the International Health Regulations focused on diseases. WHO is now responsible for providing disease-control training and expertise to countries that need such help.

New scientific evidence shows that the best way to prevent diseases from crossing borders is to make a rapid public health response at the sources of diseases. Public health measures applied at international shipping ports, international airports, and border crossings can further reduce the risk of disease spread. The 2005 regulations seek to increase protections at national borders without making unnecessary or excessive restrictions on trade and travel.

The 2005 rules provide countries with immediate guidance on how to assess, respond, and control public health risks as they arise. During an international public health emergency, WHO may recommend short-term measures that affect or restrict international trade or travel. For example, it may advise a country to require travelers arriving at its borders to undergo a basic health examination or present proof of vaccination against a specific disease.

Member State Obligations

The 2005 regulations require countries to notify WHO about any event within their borders that may be a Public Health Emergency of International Concern (PHEIC). Countries must also respond to WHO requests asking for verification of information about these events. These two rules enhance information sharing between member nations and WHO. They also help the organization to ensure effective international collaboration to prevent public health emergencies or to contain outbreaks. In many cases, WHO will inform other countries affected by the specific public health event.

WHO's efforts in support of the International Health Regulations have increased the understanding in countries of the importance of early notification of outbreaks or events. Member states have become more willing to contact WHO when a possible PHEIC is suspected. They know that they will receive timely assistance from WHO and other organizations and nations.

Under the International Health Regulations, countries must notify WHO within 24 hours in the event of a PHEIC, which is a significant public health event that meets two standards. It must constitute a public health risk to other countries through the international spread of disease, and it must have the potential to require a coordinated international response. Several factors determine whether a public health event is a PHEIC. The issues involved are:

- How severe is the potential public impact?
- Where and when is the event occurring?
- How close is the event to an international border?
- How quickly will the disease spread?
- How is the disease transmitted?
- How severe would potential restrictions to travel and trade be?

Examples of events that may constitute a PHEIC are outbreaks of pneumonic plague, West Nile fever, meningitis, and significant chemical or radiological accidents.

Through the PHEIC program, WHO can provide the world with timely notifications of serious public health events. Working with the country involved, WHO can assess the risk to global public health and inform other countries of those risks. This process reduces the likelihood that a disease will spread internationally.

The 2005 regulations set up a new, more effective system of notification. Each country must have a special office dedicated to administering the new rules. These national offices must be able to respond 24 hours a day, 7 days a week to public health events within their borders. These offices have greatly improved the capability of nations to detect and respond to public health events.

To help prevent the spread of diseases between countries, WHO member nations have agreed to set up health-control measures at international borders. The International Health Regulations require countries to conduct health inspections at international seaports and airports, as well as at major

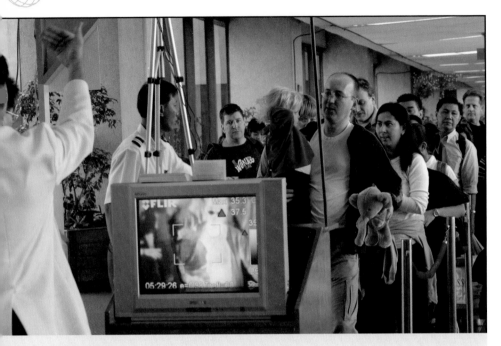

In 2003, the rapid spread of SARS in southern Asia required a quick solution at international borders. Singapore's Defense Science and Technology Agency created the thermal-imaging scanner, which reads body temperatures and detects passengers with high fevers, the most prominent symptom of SARS. The images of those with fevers show up red and these passengers are taken aside for further health checks.

ground crossings. Nations must also report to WHO any evidence of a public health risk that they have detected in other countries. A country may become aware of a risk because of potentially infected travelers or contaminated goods that either arrive at its border or have been transported abroad. For example, if a person showing symptoms of yellow fever arrives at an international airport, national health authorities will inform WHO of the person's origin. If a country discovers that cargo shipped from one of its ports may present a health risk (tainted food, for example), it must inform WHO of the ship's destinations.

By agreeing to be bound by the 2005 regulations, member nations receive several benefits. WHO provides advice and support that improves the ability of countries to detect, report, assess, and respond to public health emergencies. WHO helps low- and middle-income countries obtain the funds needed to meet their responsibilities under the regulations. WHO also provides timely, essential public-health assistance to countries that experience disease outbreaks and other serious public-health events. The organization also helps protect nations by providing up-to-date information about public-health risks worldwide.

WHO Obligations

Besides establishing obligations for WHO's member nations, the 2005 regulations also spelled out the organization's obligations. WHO must designate International Health Regulation (IHR) contacts in its country offices, regional offices, and Geneva headquarters. To detect serious public health risks, WHO must constantly monitor global public health and gather evidence about diseases worldwide. The regulations give WHO the sole authority to determine whether a particular event constitutes a PHEIC. WHO must offer technical assistance and other guidance to help nations prepare for a PHEIC within their borders. This assistance will help countries develop, strengthen, and maintain their ability to detect and respond to public health risks and emergencies. WHO also has the responsibility of updating the regulations to keep them current and based on the latest scientific knowledge. Finally, whenever a dispute involving international public health arises, the IHRs authorize WHO to negotiate a settlement between the conflicting parties.

Challenges

The 2005 regulations present many challenges to WHO and its member nations. Both WHO and the countries need adequate budgets and staff to implement the required programs. WHO's major ongoing challenge is to help lower-income countries develop the technical capacities to fulfill their obligations. Many countries lack the ability to detect and report new diseases or events at the primary health-care level. Hospitals and medical specialists in many countries also lack the ability to confirm a diagnosis of some infectious diseases, and many national health agencies do not have the means to carry out appropriate measures to control the spread of infectious diseases.

EMERGENCY AND HUMANITARIAN ACTIONS

Dangerous epidemics and the emergence of new infectious diseases can occur anywhere at any time. In many cases, they overwhelm national health systems, particularly in low-income countries. They sometimes cause many deaths and threaten a country's economic and political stability. Epidemics can also spread quickly to other countries. No single country or international agency can respond effectively to these major public health emergencies. To help countries facing a potential international public health emergency, WHO has forged partnerships and created programs to ensure that the countries have immediate access to appropriate resources and health experts.

In 2005, the United Nations designated WHO as the head of the Global Health Cluster. This group of UN organizations and other international agencies coordinates the response to health crises by all parties involved in international public health. As a result of this new leadership function, WHO has strengthened its role in dealing with the health issues that arise during natural disasters, warfare, and other emergencies. It has upgraded its capacities for rapid response, recovery efforts, and emergency preparedness.

WHO's Strategic Health Operations Center is the hub of WHO's global-response efforts. During disease outbreaks and humanitarian emergencies, the center coordinates the flow of information between WHO, its international partners, and member nations. WHO created the center in 2004. It faced its

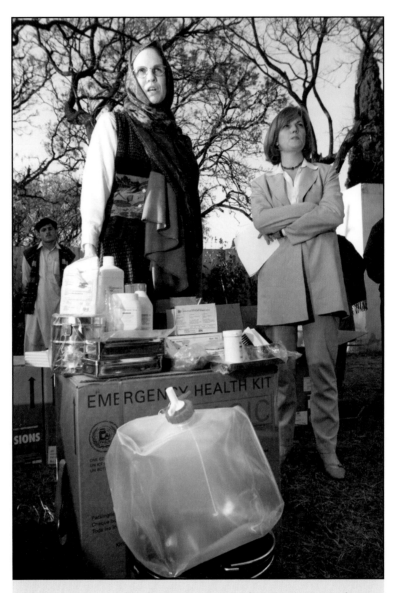

Many people in developing countries live in remote places where the nearest medical facilities are located hours or even days away from a village. People without access to basic health-care services die from preventable and treatable diseases like malaria, diarrhea, and respiratory tract infections. WHO distributes emergency health kits containing supplies and medicines that a typical population of 10,000 would need over a three-month period.

first crisis that December when a devastating tsunami struck Indonesia, Thailand, and other countries in Southeast Asia. The following year, the center coordinated the international health response to Hurricane Katrina in the United States and to an earthquake in Pakistan. The center works with three other WHO agencies to respond to international public health emergencies. It also provides advice to WHO regional and country offices, UN agencies, and international organizations on how to build emergency operation centers. It also takes part in practice exercises to prepare for global health emergencies.

The Global Outbreak Alert and Response Network

To coordinate responses to international disease outbreaks, WHO helped create the Global Outbreak Alert and Response Network in 2000. This alliance of international agencies and private enterprises helps countries control diseases by providing operational assistance. The network coordinates the delivery of medical supplies and other support to affected countries. Through the network, WHO and its partners have responded to more than 50 international disease events in more than 40 countries. They provided the assistance of more than 400 public health experts.

When faced with a potential public health emergency, the Global Outbreak Alert and Response Network investigates the event and determines whether it is likely to become a threat to international health. If the network decides that international action is needed, it assigns a project manager to coordinate the response. The project manager makes sure that appropriate assistance reaches the affected country rapidly. For example, when the SARS epidemic struck in 2003, the network assembled and sent an international team to China and Vietnam. The team included experts in respiratory diseases and epidemiology. The network worked with many partners to respond to the crisis. The U.S. Centers for Disease Control and Prevention, the United Kingdom's Public Health Laboratory Service, Australia's

Biosecurity Cooperative Research Center, Germany's Robert Koch Institute, and the nonprofit group Médecins Sans Frontières (Doctors Without Borders) were among the organizations that worked with WHO to deal with the epidemic.

In 2008, the network responded to a wide range of public health emergencies worldwide. These included:

- bird flu outbreaks in China, Indonesia, Vietnam, Pakistan, Bangladesh, and Egypt.
- Rift Valley fever outbreaks in Sudan and Madagascar.
- yellow fever outbreaks in Brazil, Paraguay, Guinea, the Ivory Coast, Burkina Faso, Central African Republic, and Liberia.
- a dengue fever outbreak in Brazil.
- an enterovirus outbreak in China.
- a polio outbreak in Nigeria.
- cholera outbreaks in Iraq and Guinea Bissau.
- a melamine-contaminated powdered infant formula crisis in China.
- a previously unknown virus in the *Arenaviridae* family in South Africa and Zambia.

To prepare in advance for public health emergencies, the Global Outbreak Alert and Response Network has created a set of emergency-response procedures. These include standards on managing the flow of information, supplies, and other resources for field teams. The network also helps countries build up health systems to prepare in advance for epidemics. These measures include establishing medical laboratories, setting up early warning systems for infectious diseases common in the country, and starting training programs.

Health Action in Crises

Natural and political crises threaten the lives and health of millions of people worldwide. These crises include earthquakes, hurricanes, wars, and civil unrest. WHO's Health Action in Crises program works with international partners and member countries to help local communities respond to and recover from humanitarian emergencies. Emergencies of this magnitude often overwhelm local and national health systems, particularly in developing countries. The primary goal of Health

WHO REACTS TO A HUMANITARIAN CRISIS

On May 2, 2008, a powerful cyclone struck the nation of Myanmar (formerly Burma). Cyclone Nargis slashed through Yangon, the nation's largest city, and the country's low-lying delta region. High winds and widespread flooding left more than 150,000 people dead or missing. The worst natural catastrophe in Myanmar's history disrupted the lives of as many as 2.5 million people. Twelve-year-old Leh Ler Shee survived by clinging to a tree after a surge of water destroyed the house he was in. He recalled, "I saw many dead bodies, dead cattle, and debris everywhere. I went back home and saw that my house had collapsed. I tried to find my mother but I couldn't."*

The World Health Organization immediately sprang into action. Its country office in Yangon handled the initial response. The Health Action in Crises program and WHO's Southeast Asia Regional Office coordinated efforts to send supplies and emergency-response teams to the devastated country. More than 140 WHO staff members soon arrived to assess the public health situation and to help coordinate the health response. With the support of Italy, Health Action in Crises provided 10 emergency health kits, which had enough supplies to provide essential care to 300,000 people for three months. WHO and the governments of Norway and Denmark donated nearly $500,000 to buy urgently needed medical supplies.

Action in Crises is to lower the number of deaths, reduce the amount of suffering, and ensure the health of populations.

When a crisis occurs, Health Action in Crises works with the UN Executive Committee on Humanitarian Affairs and the UN humanitarian coordinator assigned to the event. The coordinator oversees the humanitarian efforts of WHO and other

The storm destroyed health-care facilities and medications and killed or dislocated health-care workers. As survivors fled the still-submerged delta region, overcrowding and the lack of safe water and adequate sanitation facilities posed a severe threat to public health. WHO officials became concerned about the risk of infectious diseases— particularly cholera, malaria, and tuberculosis—spreading through the country.

Worries about epidemics soon faded. Only a few dozen cases of dengue fever and higher-than-normal levels of diarrheal diseases were reported. Richard Garfield of the Health and Nutrition Tracking Service, an international partnership hosted by Health Action in Crises, observed, "The most important thing that . . . WHO took part in was an assessment of the needs in the region, visiting 291 villages throughout this very remote region. . . . We have never had this kind of assessment after a major disaster, so we know now what the needs are and how they have changed since the disaster."[**]

* Nattha Kennapan, "Child-Friendly Spaces Provide Refuge for Cyclone-Affected Children in Myanmar," UNICEF. June 5, 2008. Available online at *www.unicef.org/infobycountry/myanmar_44377.html*.

** Transcript of WHO podcast, July 28, 2008. Available online at *www.who.int/mediacentre/multimedia/podcasts/2008/transcript_40/en/index.html*.

international organizations. Health Action in Crises makes sure that there is an adequate response to health issues during the crisis. Following the crisis, the program helps the country rebuild its health systems and advises on how to maintain those systems. It also helps countries improve their ability to respond to future disasters. Funds for the program's activities come from the World Health Assembly and the UN's Central Emergency Response Fund.

In 2008, Health Action in Crises helped supply emergency medicine and equipment to victims of a flood that struck India and Nepal. More than 3.4 million people were affected when the waters of the Kosi River overflowed its banks. Samlee Plianbangchang, WHO's regional director for Southeast Asia, noted, "WHO's assistance includes supplying emergency medicines and equipment for 180,000 people, supporting disease surveillance and child immunization campaigns and ensuring safe drinking water."[16]

Program on Disease Control in Humanitarian Emergencies

WHO's program on Disease Control in Humanitarian Emergencies responds to humanitarian emergencies in which large numbers of people have been displaced. When natural disasters strike, people often move temporarily to places that are unable to handle the influx of people. Inadequate food and shelter, unsafe drinking water, and poor sanitation often increase the risk of the spread of infectious diseases. Health officials can encounter high rates of respiratory infections, diarrheal diseases, and infectious diseases like measles, malaria, and tuberculosis.

The program works to reduce the effects of diseases during humanitarian emergencies and in longer crises, such as civil wars. Its major focus is to provide technical and operational support to Health Action in Crises, WHO regional and country offices, national heath-care agencies, and other UN and international agencies. It develops guidelines for controlling communicable diseases during humanitarian crises. The program works to strengthen international and local partnerships to be better prepared for such crises. In 2008, it provided support to protect the health of populations in 12 conflict-torn countries, including Afghanistan, Chad, Liberia, Somalia, and Sudan.

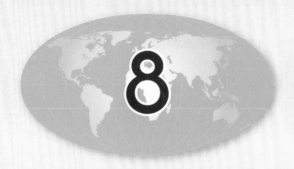

8

Health Care for Everyone

In 2008, WHO celebrated its sixtieth anniversary. To chronicle its history since 1948, the organization produced books, videos, and podcasts and sponsored photo exhibits, seminars, and other events. All of these activities showed the significant impact of WHO's efforts over the decades to improve global public health. The organization also used the milestone to draw attention to the important challenges that the organization continues to face and its plans to meet those challenges in the future.

WHO has achieved many notable successes, such as the eradication of smallpox, its rapid responses to countless epidemics, and its effective programs that prevent polio, measles, and other diseases. Its efforts to improve underlying factors that affect health—such as the environment, diet and nutrition, and tobacco control—have achieved mixed results. These undertakings have obligated the organization to deal with such complex issues as poverty, globalization, human rights, and social justice.

WHO remains the world's foremost source of public health information. It shares its scientific, technical, training, and administrative knowledge with its member nations and other international organizations. These efforts help member nations to prevent, treat, and cure diseases and other threats to public health. WHO works to prevent epidemics, respond to public health emergencies, and assist in achieving the UN's Millennium Development Goals. It sponsors public health conferences, publications, and outreach programs. Perhaps most importantly, as two public health scholars have noted, WHO is the "world's health conscience."[17] It serves as an advocate for the poor and the powerless who desperately need health care. It seeks to ensure that everyone in the world has access to quality health care.

WHO's efforts to improve health around the world involve more than employing medical science and public health policy. Its work touches on issues of economics, politics, environmentalism, and culture. Perhaps the most difficult challenges facing global public health—and, therefore, WHO—is poverty. Roughly 6.7 billion people now inhabit the planet. More than 2.5 billion of them live on less than $2 a day. They struggle to pay for food, clothing, shelter, and other essentials. Many of the world's poor receive little or no health care.

More than half of the world's nations are developing countries. Poor nutrition, unsafe drinking water, and inadequate sanitation are common problems in these countries. These conditions often lead to high rates of disease and death. Many developing countries lack the financial means to build and sustain adequate national health systems. These nations suffer from a shortage of medicines and a lack of technology

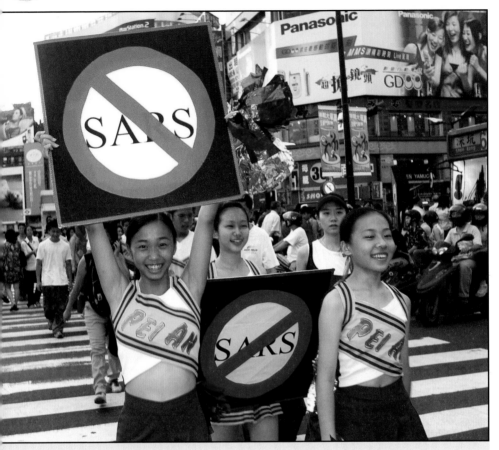

Outbreaks of emerging and epidemic-prone diseases are increasing, due to rapid urbanization, environmental mismanagement, the trading of food, and the misuse of antibiotics. WHO has answered the world's call to collectively defend itself against health security threats and participates in reforms to improve its efficiency and effectiveness so that all people have access to basic health services. Above, a cheer team participates in a rally celebrating Taiwan's removal from the SARS affected-area list by WHO in July 2003.

and other medical equipment. Many also have too few or poorly trained health-care workers. Poverty and health often link together in a downward spiral. Poor public health results in less economic output and lower national incomes. Low national incomes hinder countries in building and maintaining adequate health-care systems. Improving health in developing countries can improve their ability to expand their economies and strengthen their health-care systems. Strong health-care systems will produce healthier citizens who can work, attend school, and create more prosperous lives for themselves.

WHO also faces several organizational challenges. The public health needs of WHO's member nations vary greatly. These differences have created a rift between low- to middle-income members and high-income members. Developing countries want WHO to address their health needs, particularly the strengthening of primary health-care systems and the improvement of access to affordable medications and medical technologies. Wealthier members have questioned the appropriateness of WHO adopting these roles.

In carrying out its mission, WHO has also become increasingly dependent on outside groups. It works with other UN agencies and a wide range of international nongovernmental organizations to develop global public health research, policies, and programs. WHO now relies less on funding from member nations and more on funding from corporations and charitable foundations. The need to collaborate with other organizations expands WHO's reach and improves its effectiveness. It also weakens its independence and neutrality and slows its response to health issues.

WHO faces many health-related challenges. The threat of new diseases, such as Ebola and SARS, remains a constant concern. New strains of known infectious diseases have also emerged. Many are resistant to the drugs commonly used to treat the disease, making uncontrollable epidemics a continuing threat. Drug companies are developing few antibiotics to battle infections. Instead, they are focusing their research and development on more profitable products, such as drugs to treat symptoms of chronic diseases and nonessential medications to treat conditions like baldness.

Lifestyle changes in developing countries, with people consuming foods higher in sugar and fat and using more tobacco products, have increased health risks in those countries. Armed conflicts and natural disasters interfere with WHO programs and lead to epidemics and other health problems. The growth of threats to healthy environments, such as pollution and global warming, threaten the well-being of people worldwide.

WHO staff in a wide range of departments, programs, and teams work around the world to improve global health. WHO microbiologists monitor changes in virus subtypes. WHO doctors help develop new drugs. WHO researchers study links between health and diet. Employees at WHO country offices deliver vaccines to war-torn regions. These are only a few of the people at WHO striving to make the world healthier.

Since its inception, WHO has earned an excellent international reputation. It makes a unique contribution to global public health and the lives of people worldwide. In carrying out its mission to achieve "the attainment by all peoples of the highest possible level of health,"[18] WHO will continue to strengthen the world's united defense against epidemics and other risks that threaten global public health. It will continue to help countries build and sustain national health-care systems. In 2008, Margaret Chan, WHO's director-general, reasserted the organization's resolve to continue to advocate for fair access to essential health care. She declared, "Health systems will not automatically gravitate towards greater fairness and efficiency. . . . Our world will not become a fair place for health all by itself."[19] All of WHO's efforts will continue to be based on the belief that all human life matters and that everyone deserves good health.

CHRONOLOGY

1300s   Venice quarantines visitors and vessels from abroad.

1830s   The first sanitary board is founded in Alexandria, Egypt.

1851   The first international sanitary conference is held in Paris, France.

1892   The first international sanitary rules are approved.

1902   The world's first global health organization, the International Sanitary Bureau, is founded.

1918   A global campaign to eradicate yellow fever is launched.

1920   The Health Organization of the League of Nations is founded.

1946   The United Nations Economic and Social Council proposes a specialized UN agency for health.

1948   The World Health Organization begins its operations.

The first World Health Assembly is held.

1951   New International Sanitary Regulations are adopted.

1959   The first *World Health Situation Report* is published.

1969   International Sanitary Regulations are revised and renamed the International Health Regulations.

1977   The World Health Assembly adopts Health for All by the Year 2000 resolution.

1980   WHO announces the eradication of smallpox.

1987   The Global Program on AIDS is created.

1995   The first *World Health Report* is published.

WHO launches its DOTS strategy for tuberculosis.

2000   WHO establishes the Global Outbreak Alert and Response Network.

The UN adopts Millennium Development Goals.

2003   The World Health Assembly adopts the Framework Convention on Tobacco Control.

WHO coordinates the international response to the SARS outbreak.

2004   The World Health Assembly adopts the Global Strategy on Diet, Physical Activity, and Health.

2005   International Health Regulations are substantially revised.

2008   WHO celebrates its sixtieth anniversary.

NOTES

Introduction

1. "SARS Outbreak Contained Worldwide." WHO press release, July 5, 2003. Available online at *www.who.int/mediacentre/news/releases/2003/pr56/en/*.

Chapter 1

2. Constitution of the World Health Organization. Available online at *www.who.int/governance/eb/constitution/en/index.html*.
3. UN Office for the Coordination of Humanitarian Affairs, Integrated Regional Information Networks. "AFRICA: Low Cost Meningitis Vaccine Developed," March 4, 2008. Available online at *www.irinnews.org/report.aspx?ReportID=77105*.
4. World Health Organization. *Working for Health: An Introduction to the World Health Organization*. Geneva, Switzerland: WHO Press, 2007, p. 7. Available online at *www.who.int/about/brochure_en.pdf*.

Chapter 2

5. Paul De Kruif, *Microbe Hunters*. New York: Harcourt, 2002, p. 92.
6. UN General Assembly, *Prevention and Control of Acquired Immunodeficiency Syndrome (AIDS)*, Resolution 42/8 (1987).

Chapter 3

7. World Health Organization. *Working for Health: An Introduction to the World Health Organization*. Geneva, Switzerland: WHO Press, 2007, p. 7. Available online at *www.who.int/about/brochure_en.pdf*.

Chapter 4

8.   UN General Assembly. *United Nations Millennium Declaration*, September 9, 2000.

9.   WHO/UNICEF. *Global Plan for Reducing Measles Mortality 2006–2010*. Geneva, Switzerland: World Health Organization, 2006, p. 2.

10.   World Health Organization. *Health-Promoting Schools: A Healthy Setting for Living, Learning, and Working*. Geneva, Switzerland: World Health Organization, 1998, p. 6. Available online at *www.who.int/school_youth_health/media/en/92.pdf*.

11.   World Health Organization—Gender, Women, and Health Program. "Integrating Gender Analysis and Actions into the Work of WHO." Available online at *www.who.int/gender/mainstreaming/integrating_gender/en/index.html*.

Chapter 5

12.   Stop TB Partnership. "Bam! Kapow! Figo Scores a Goal Against Tuberculosis in a New Comic Book," July 24, 2008. Available online at *www.stoptb.org/figo/News.asp*.

Chapter 6

13.   World Health Organization. *World Health Statistics 2008*. Geneva, Switzerland: World Health Organization, 2008, p. 29.

14.   World Health Organization. *Fight Against Cancer: Strategies That Prevent, Cure, and Care*. Geneva, Switzerland: World Health Organization, 2007, p. 4.

15.   World Health Organization. *WHO Report on the Global Tobacco Epidemic*. Geneva, Switzerland: World Health Organization, 2008, p. 7.

Chapter 7

16. "WHO Chips in to Help Flood Victims in Bihar." *Times of India*, September 6, 2008. Available online at *timesofindia. indiatimes.com/articleshow/msid-3453223,prtpage-1.cms*.

Chapter 8

17. Kent Buse and Gill Walt, "Globalisation and Multilateral Public-Private Health Partnerships: Issues for Health Policy" in *Health Policy in a Globalizing World*, Kelley Lee, ed. New York: Cambridge University Press, 2002, p. 56.

18. Constitution of the World Health Organization. Available online at *www.who.int/governance/eb/constitution/ en/index.html*.

19. Margaret Chan, "Global Action to Strengthen Health Systems," keynote address at the G8 Tokyo summit, November 3, 2008. Available online at *www.who.int/dg/ speeches/2008/20081103/en/index.html*.

BIBLIOGRAPHY

Asia Pacific Leadership Forum on HIV/AIDS and Development. *Portraits of Commitment: Why People Become Leaders in AIDS Work.* Bangkok, Thailand: Asia Pacific Leadership Forum on HIV/AIDS and Development, 2007. Available online. URL: http://www.aplfaids.com/documents/SA_Portraits_book.pdf.

Breslow, Lester et al., eds. *The Encyclopedia of Public Health.* New York: Macmillan, 2001.

Burci, Gian Luca and Claude-Henri Vignes. *World Health Organization.* The Hague, The Netherlands: Kluwer Law International, 2004.

Buse, Kent and Gill Walt. "Globalisation and Multilateral Public-Private Health Partnerships: Issues for Health Policy" in *Health Policy in a Globalizing World*, Kelley Lee, ed. New York: Cambridge University Press, 2002.

Chan, Margaret. "Global Action to Strengthen Health Systems," keynote address at the G8 Tokyo summit, November 3, 2008. Available online. URL: http://www.who.int/dg/speeches/2008/20081103/en/index.html.

De Kruif, Paul. *Microbe Hunters.* New York: Harcourt, 2002.

Fidler, David R. "The Globalization of Public Health: The First 100 Years of International Health Diplomacy" in *Bulletin of the World Health Organization.* Geneva, Switzerland: World Health Organization, 2001.

Jaret, Peter. *Impact: Dispatches from the Front Lines of Global Health.* Washington, D.C.: National Geographic, 2003.

Kennapan, Nattha. "Child-Friendly Spaces Provide Refuge for Cyclone-Affected Children in Myanmar," UNICEF. June 5, 2008. Available online. URL: http://www.unicef.org/infobycountry/myanmar_44377.html.

Lee, Kelley. *Historical Dictionary of the World Health Organization.* Lanham, Md.: Scarecrow Press, 1998.

———. *World Health Organization*. New York: Routledge, 2008.

Lerner, K. Lee and Brenda Wilmoth Lerner, eds. *World of Microbiology and Immunology*. Farmington Hills, Mich.: Gale, 2002.

Piddock, Charles. *Outbreaks: Science Seeks Safeguards for Global Health*. Washington, D.C.: National Geographic, 2008.

"SARS Outbreak Contained Worldwide." WHO press release, July 5, 2003. Available online. URL: http://www.who.int/mediacentre/news/releases/2003/pr56/en/.

Sixty-First World Health Assembly. Agenda item 11.10, WHA61.4., May 24, 2008, "Strategies to Reduce the Harmful Use of Alcohol." Available online. URL: http://www.who.int/nmh/WHA%2061.4.pdf.

Stop TB Partnership. "Bam! Kapow! Figo Scores a Goal Against Tuberculosis in a New Comic Book,." Press release dated July 24, 2008. Available online. URL: http://www.stoptb.org/figo/News.asp.

Tibayrenc, Michel. *Encyclopedia of Infectious Diseases*. Hoboken, N.J.: Wiley, 2007.

Transcript of WHO podcast, July 28, 2008. Available online. URL: http://www.who.int/mediacentre/multimedia/podcasts/2008/transcript_40/en/index.html.

United Nations. *The Millennium Development Goals Update 2008*. New York: United Nations, 2008.

United Nations Department of Economic and Social Affairs. *The Millennium Development Goals Report 2006*. New York: United Nations, 2006.

United Nations General Assembly. *United Nations Millennium Declaration*, September 9, 2000.

———. *Prevention and Control of Acquired Immunodeficiency Syndrome (AIDS)*, Resolution 42/8, October 26, 1987.

United Nations Office for the Coordination of Humanitarian Affairs, Integrated Regional Information Networks. "AFRICA: Low Cost Meningitis Vaccine Developed," March 4, 2008. Available online. URL: http://www.irinnews.org/report.aspx?ReportID=77105.

"WHO Chips in to Help Flood Victims in Bihar." *Times of India*, September 6, 2008. Available online. URL: http://timesofindia.indiatimes.com/articleshow/msid-3453223,prtpage-1.cms.

Wide Angle: Birth of a Surgeon: Aaron Brown Interview: Dr. Margaret Chan. PBS. Available online. URL: http://www.pbs.org/wnet/wideangle/episodes/birth-of-a-surgeon/aaron-brown-interview-dr-margaret-chan/1810/.

Wide Angle: Birth of a Surgeon—Midwives in Mozambique. PBS. Available online. URL: http://www.pbs.org/wnet/wideangle/episodes/birth-of-a-surgeon/introduction/747/.

World Health Organization. Constitution of the World Health Organization. Available online. URL: http://www.who.int/governance/eb/constitution/en/index.html.

———. *Fight Against Cancer: Strategies That Prevent, Cure, and Care.* Geneva, Switzerland: World Health Organization, 2007.

———. Gender, Women, and Health Program. "Integrating Gender Analysis and Actions into the Work of WHO." Available online. URL: http://www.who.int/gender/mainstreaming/integrating_gender/en/index.html.

———. *Health-Promoting Schools: A Healthy Setting for Living, Learning, and Working.* Geneva, Switzerland: World Health Organization, 1998. Available online. URL: http://www.who.int/school_youth_health/media/en/92.pdf.

———. *WHO Report on the Global Tobacco Epidemic.* Geneva, Switzerland: World Health Organization, 2008.

———. *Working for Health: An Introduction to the World Health Organization.* Geneva, Switzerland: WHO Press, 2007.

———. *World Health Report 2008.* Geneva, Switzerland: World Health Organization, 2008.

———. *World Health Statistics 2008.* Geneva, Switzerland: World Health Organization, 2008.

WHO/UNICEF. *Global Plan for Reducing Measles Mortality 2006–2010.* Geneva, Switzerland: World Health Organization, 2006,

FURTHER READING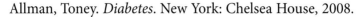

Allman, Toney. *Diabetes*. New York: Chelsea House, 2008.

Beck-Sague, Consuelo and Caridad Beck. *HIV/AIDS*. New York: Chelsea House, 2003.

Bookmiller, Kirsten Nakjavani. *The United Nations*. New York: Chelsea House, 2008.

Bozzone, Donna M. *Causes of Cancer*. New York: Chelsea House, 2007.

Coleman, William. *Cholera*. New York: Chelsea House, 2008.

Emmeluth, Donald. *Influenza*. New York: Chelsea House, 2008.

Finer, Kim Renee. *Tuberculosis*. New York: Chelsea House, 2003.

———. *Smallpox*. New York: Chelsea House, 2004.

Hinds, Maurene J. *Fighting the AIDS and HIV Epidemic: A Global Battle*. Berkeley Heights, N.J.: Enslow Publishers, 2007.

Marcus, Bernard A. *Malaria*. New York: Chelsea House, 2003.

Senker, Cath. *World Health Organization*. Chicago: Raintree, 2004.

Serradell, Joaquima. *SARS*. New York: Chelsea House, 2003.

Turkington, Carol and Bonnie Lee Ashby. *The Encyclopedia of Infectious Diseases*. New York: Facts on File, 2007.

Youngerman, Barry. *Pandemics and Global Health*. New York: Facts on File, 2008.

WEB SITES

Centers for Disease Control and Prevention
http://www.cdc.gov

This site provides reliable, up-to-date health information for individuals, public health professionals, health-care providers, researchers and scientists, policy makers, students, etc.

Roll Back Malaria Partnership
http://www.rollbackmalaria.org

Campaign launched in 1998 by WHO, UNICEF, the UN Development Program, and the World Bank to provide a global coordinated approach to fighting malaria.

Stop TB Partnership
http://www.stoptb.org

Established in 2000 to realize the goal of eliminating tuberculosis as a public health problem.

The United Nations
http://www.un.org.

International organization that facilitates cooperation in international law, international security, economic development, social progress, human rights, and achieving world peace.

The World Bank
http://www.worldbank.org

A bank that provides financial and technical assistance to developing countries for development programs (bridges, roads, schools) with the goal of reducing poverty.

UNAIDS (Joint United Nations Program on HIV/AIDS)
http://www.unaids.org

Joint venture of the United Nations members to help the world prevent new HIV infections, care for people living with HIV, and lessen the impact of the epidemic.

UNICEF (United Nations Children's Fund)
http://www.unicef.org.

Global organization that provides long-term humanitarian and development assistance to children and mothers in developing countries.

World Health Organization
http://www.who.int

A specialized agency of the United Nations that acts as the authority on health.

PICTURE CREDITS

INDEX

ABOUT THE CONTRIBUTORS

G. S. PRENTZAS is the author of more than 20 books for young readers. He is the author of *Gideon v. Wainwright* in Chelsea House's GREAT SUPREME COURT DECISIONS series and *The Brooklyn Bridge* in Chelsea House's BUILDING AMERICA THEN AND NOW series. He has also written books on law, government, geography, and history, covering such topics as the right to counsel, criminal rights, Native American law, and the FBI.

Series editor **PEGGY KAHN** is professor of political science at the University of Michigan-Flint. She teaches courses in European politics, lived in England for many years, and has written about British politics. She has been a social studies volunteer in the Ann Arbor public schools. Her Ph.D. in political science is from the University of California, Berkeley, and her B.A. in history and government is from Oberlin College.